VATA VYADHI

VATA VYADHI

(PAKSHAGHATA)
(HEMIPLEGIA)

DR. B.G. GOPINATH

B.A. D.S.A.C, H.P.A. (Jamnagar)
Former Professor and Head
Postgraduate Dept. of Kayachikitsa
Government Ayurveda Medical College, Mysuru

SINCE 1903

MOTILAL BANARSIDASS
PUBLISHING HOUSE

*First Edition: Delhi, **2025***

Also available at:

MOTILAL BANARSIDASS PUBLISHING HOUSE

- 4637/20, F-2, Hari Sadan, First Floor, Ansari Road, Darya Ganj Delhi–110 002 *Tel.*: (+91-11) 4559 7999
- 1st Floor, 1/2 Rathnavilas Road, Basvanagudi, Next to Pai Vista Convention Hall, South End Circle, Bengaluru–560004 (India) *Tel.*: +91-80-41275911

ISBN: 978-93-6853-622-2 (Hardcover)
ISBN: 978-93-6853-270-5 (Paperback)

Printed & Published by
Rajendra P Jain *for*
Motilal Banarsidass Publishing House
A-44, Naraina Industrial Area, Phase I, New Delhi–110 028 (INDIA)
Email: naraina@mlbd.in Website: www.mlbd.in
Tel.: (+91-11) 4751 1592

DEDICATION

Dedicated to the lotus feet of my venerated father proficient in spiritual discourses, pious gem, gem of a physician Sri Ganesha Subraya Patela who guided me through my childhood in gaining a positive interest in Indian culture, tradition, knowledge and wisdom.

Contents

PREFACE

Yo vishwam vidadhati pati satatam samharayatyanjasa
Srishtva divyamahoushadheemscha vividhan doorikarotyamayan
Bibhranonjalina chakasti bhuvanam peeyusha purnam ghatam
Tam dhanvantarirupameeshamamalam vandamahe shreyase//

It is our good fortune that ancient Sanskrit manuscripts written on various topics of Ayurveda are accessible in plenty even today. However it is our misfortune that since they are in Sanskrit which is not propagated to that extent in our country and they are in the form of aphorisms, many among us do not have the competence to understand them in totality. This is particularly applicable to the present-day student community. The present-day students have adequate intellectual competence. Many among them have a thirst for knowledge. There is a dearth of literature that can quench their thirst. Hence to compile the subject matter contained in ancient texts deliberated in a manner appropriate to the current epoch is one among the present-day exigencies.

Even though classics contain a detailed description of many diseases, the nidana panchaka (fivefold diagnostic factors) along with upadrava (supervenient afflictions), sadhyasadhyata (prognosis) and chikitsatmaka varnana (therapeutic description) have been narrated very briefly. Even though the nidana panchaka (fivefold diagnostic factors), sadhyasadhyata (prognosis) and chikitsa (treatment) pertaining to a multitude of diseases coming under one category have been commonly narrated, each disease categorized under that group has not been individually described with regard to the nidana panchaka (fivefold diagnostic factors).

Modern Ayurveda scholars such as Dr.Yadavaji trikamaji acharya, Dr. R.R. Pathak, Dr. R.R Desai, etc have written in extensive detail and deliberation on only those diseases whose nidana panchaka (fivefold diagnostic factors), etc are described in detail in the classics. It appears that in none of the Indian languages is there a detailed description based on nidana panchaka (fivefold diagnostic factors) of individual diseases that are described briefly under whatever categorization; the disease that can be specifically named in this group is Vatavyadhis. Specialized individual description of each of the diseases such as Grdrasi, Apabahuka, Akshepaka, Pakshaghata, etc coming under this group cannot be beholden.

Hence assuming that it is essential to write about Vatavyadhi in the same style as delineated by the afore-mentioned scholars, this book has been written.

While narrating the names of rishis (sages) in Kautilya Arthashastra there is reference to a sage "Vatavyadhi" at one place. The renowned commentator of this text in 'Jayamangala teeka' implies Vatavyadhi as Udhava muni (Kau. A. sha. Amatyotpatti chapter). There is no relationship between this sage and Vatavyadhi of Ayurveda. Here Vatavyadhi means a category of multiple diseases caused by Vata.

Pakshaghata, a cardinal disease belonging to this classification has been narrated in detail in the present text. In the first chapter the importance of Vatavyadhi has been indicated and how complex they are and subsequently classification has been given so as to facilitate their study. As to which of the disease in modern medicine resembles Pakshaghata has been narrated giving justifications.

A history of this disease has been narrated in the second chapter after deliberating, as far as possible, on writings starting from Vedic literature to all published important Ayurveda literature available to this day. In this, latest therapeutic drugs acting against the disease resorted to at different epochs and the progression in the line of treatment at different epochs can be identified.

The third chapter carries a detailed deliberation of paribashe (definition) of Pakshaghata, vyutpatti (etymology) and different terms carrying identical meaning [paryayanama (synonyms)].

The fourth chapter carries the narration of etiological factors of Pakshaghata. Here more emphasis has been placed on internal etiologies since specific external etiologies for Pakshaghata cannot be seen in the classics. How abscess, tumours, etc. described in modern texts can be etiological factors for Pakshaghata as per Ayurveda perspective has been deliberated with adequate corroboration. In this context one nidanartakara (etiologically relevant) disease that has remained without citing is a Sannipataja jwara (Conjunctive fever) called 'Sanjna' - where all the three doshas are involved. There is evidence that this can also cause Pakshaghata.

The samprapti (pathogenesis) has been narrated employing the principles pertaining to samprapti ghataka (components of pathogenesis) in the fifth chapter. An effort has been made to prove that the abode of the illness is one part of the brain invoking evidence from the classics. It has been said in this context that this disease is related to Vatavaha srotas (system of vata - nervous system). The Vatavaha srotas (system of vata), that is elaborated, has been depicted to have an equivalent connotation to the nervous system of modern (medicine). Vatavaha srotas (system of vata) is simply not a figment of imagination. It has been said in the Chapter 5 of Charaka vimana stana that dosha (vitiators) also have independent conduits.

Vata pitta sleshmanam punaha sarvashareeracharanam
sarvani srotamsi ayanabhutani (Cha.vi.5)

It has been presumed on this premise as Vatavaha srotas (system of vata).

A comparative appraisal of signs and symptoms enumerated in the classics with signs and symptoms given in modern science is provided in Chapter 6. Signs and symptoms have been classified as pratyatma (cardinal) or anushangika (concommitant) and each described in detail.

Differential diagnosis has been narrated in the Chapter 7 to show how diseases like Ekangavata (Monoplegia), Ardita (Bell's palsy), Pangu (Paraplegia), Khanja (a type of Monoplegia), etc are different from Pakshaghata. Signs and symptoms relevant to sadhyasadhyata (prognosis) have been sequentially compiled and recounted in tabular form. Subsequently the method of examination of the patient has been appended after emphasizing the important points to be noted to understand the nidana panchaka (fivefold diagnostic factors) vyavachedaka nidana (differential diagnosis) and sadhyasadhyata (prognosis) of this disease.

All the principles of treatment pertaining to Pakshaghata have been compiled and the type of treatment, its duration and the sequence in which it has to be done is described in Chapter 8 along with a time-bound progression. The karmukatva (functional aspect) of line of treatment has been briefly stated from the standpoint of Ayurveda. While explaining the sequence of peyadi krama (conciliatory sequence through thin gruel, etc) after shodana (purification) instead of the preponderant opinion that all patients should be given akrta yusha (unseasoned greengram soup) and akrta mamsa rasa (unseasoned mutton soup) as well as krta yusha (seasoned greengram soup) and krta mamsa rasa (seasoned mutton soup) keeping in view the religious feelings and satmya / asatmya (wholesome / unwholesome) of the patient towards food, this book has acknowledged the minority view point that akrta yusha (unseasoned greengram soup) **or** akrta mamsa rasa (unseasoned mutton soup) as well as krta yusha (seasoned greengram soup) **or** krta mamsa rasa (seasoned mutton soup) should be administered. After basti chikitsa (therapeutic enema) ahara krama (sequential diet) and chikitsa krama karmukatva (functionality of therapeutic sequence) have been narrated conforming to the rasa samsarjana krama (sequence of conciliation by savoury).

Dietary sequence correlated to therapeutic sequence indicating what diet should be given on what day has been given in tabular form in the Chapter 9. Finally, not only all the medications that are said to be employable in Pakshaghata have been given in alphabetical order based upon formulations such as taila (oils), ghrta (clarified butter), vati (pills) etc but also the table of ingredients that go into these formulations. The numbers indicated against the ingredient substance indicates that this ingredient substance has been explained in the formulations pertaining to the respective numbers. From a glance of this it can be understood that an ingredient substance is present in all the formulations of all the numbers denoted in front. Only those formulations have been chosen and expounded here where the term Pakshaghata or its synonym has been used while narrating the qualities of the formulation in the classics.

On the whole a sincere effort has been made to give this book a comprehensive consummate literary image. This is the maiden literary efflorescence of the author "the first part of a literary series called 'Vatavyadhi". There is a desire to write in as much detail about other diseases of Vata like Pangu (Paraplegia), Khanja (a form of Monoplegia), Apabahuka (Adhesive capsulitis), Akshepaka (Convulsions), etc. in the second part. There is a desire to place the second part in the hands of the readers as early as possible through the encouragement of the students and community of physicians as well as the grace of Dhanvantari.

It is not an exaggeration to state that when the draft was prepared there was neither the intention to print and publish it nor the conviction. I am extremely grateful to my confident and beloved of all Dr. S. M. Angadi, Principal, Government Ayurveda Medical College, Mysuru, who himself is a scholar, for not only reading this draft, providing pertinent suggestions and encouraged entreatingly to print and publish but also for writing the prelude. I cannot but remember my affable colleagues as well as Asst.Professor Dr. M. Eshwar Reddy for their incessant endeavours along with me, from the point of preparation of the draft of this book to the point of printing and for convincing me that publication of such a book is very essential for the student community and also for providing the help of other patrons in aid of printing. Heartfelt gratefulness to students of BAMS Sri Jayavanth, Ms. Nagarathna, Ms Vanishri and Ms.Sudha who assisted in preparing the table of ingredients of compound formulations useful in Pakshaghata as well as to Dr. Vasanta, lecturer of this college who toiled and assisted in the prevention of repetition of the same drug multiple times in the table.

I am infinitely indebted to Sri. Govindappa Shetty who provided financial assistance in printing and also sent his best wishes, Sri Shankar, proprietor of Sri Bhuvaneshwari printers who methodically and precisely printed and supplied at the right time, Sri Ganesh gudi artist, owners of Ravi block makers, Sri B.G. Chakrapani Rao, owner of Sri. Barige Rameshwara publishers who agreed to publish this book, authors of the texts referred by myself in writing this book, Dr. Swarna Prasad of Sri Datta Ayurvedalaya who assisted me continuously in making corrections to the printed draft and to students as well as colleagues who directly or indirectly cooperated.

In Spite of utmost care, I regret inability to prevent the onslaught of printers' devil.

Bhishajam sadhu vrittanam bhadramagama shalinam/
abhyastakarmanam bhadram bhadram bhadrabhilashinam//

PREFACE

It gives me immense pleasure to place this English version of my book 'Vatavyadhi' (Pakshaghata) written in Kannada about three and a half decades ago, which actually became out of print just a year after its publication. Soon after there was a demand from students, teachers and the other Ayurveda fraternity, especially from states outside Karnataka and also students of Ayurveda colleges in Karnataka who were from other states, to bring out this book in English. I too felt the demand was genuine. Since then, it was my cherished desire to bring out an English version of it in order to quench the thirst of knowledge of the younger generations. However, on account of my pre-occupations, serious health hazards beyond my control and also advanced age, I could not make my dream come true for decades. But then destiny wished it to happen and thus it happened. One day my friend and junior colleague Dr. M. Ramesh, a retired Professor from Government Ayurveda Medical College, Bengaluru, contacted me over the phone to enquire about my health. It was certainly a pleasant surprise to me. After preliminary conversations, the matter of translating my book in Kannada to English, which was relegated to the background for a long time, came up and he voluntarily opted to take up this ' not so easy job'. My joy knew no bounds to learn this and eventually I gave my heart felt consent on the spot. Dr.Ramesh worked with full devotion and dedication consequent to which this English version of my book is made available to all interested readers so that the knowledge stream can continue to flow for years to come. I regret for not being able to cover all Vatavyadhi's, though initially intended to. Vatavyadhi's are stated to be more than eighty in number, each one of them or quite a few of them are major diseases like Grdhrasi, Vishvachi, Antarayama, Bahirayama, Manyastambha, Apabahuka, Ardhita, Pangu, Udavarta, Aanaha, Aadmana and so on and so forth need to be covered in detail in so far as their diagnostic and therapeutic dimensions are concerned, on the same lines as this book. However if the present translated work motivates younger generations to think and act in this direction so as to keep our precious knowledge and heritage ever growing and glittering, the effort put in here will be really worth it. I hope and trust that my humble desire will fructify in the near future.

Lastly I remain thankful to Dr. M. Ramesh for his great service and pray that Lord Dhanvantari should bestow him with extremely good health, a long and happy wholesome life.

Bengaluru
August 25, 2023

Dr. B.G.Gopinath
Former Dean
Sri Sri College of Ayurveda
Bengaluru.

Foreword

Dr. B. G. Gopinath who wrote and brought out this excellent book by name Vatavyadhi (Pakshaghata-Hemiplegia) has made an in-depth study of the science of Ayurveda and by his outstanding teaching has earned appreciation of undergraduate and postgraduate students as well as all of us. When viewed compared to other states of India, those who have authored literary works relevant to Ayurveda in Karnataka and in Kannada are meagre. That too those who have written this type of book are very rare. Though there are many among us, who are competent in writing, they are not coming forward since they have insufficient encouragement.

We became known to each other for the first time, when we gained admission, together, for the postgraduate course (HPA) in Jamnagar, Gujarat. Our stay together in the same room of the hostel there led to greater affinity. That was a time of excellent opportunity for us to discuss every day different aspects of the science.

Vatavyadhi is among the eight major diseases (Mahavyadhi). Even amidst them Pakshaghata (Hemiplegia) is a formidable and difficult to treat disease. Many are succumbing to this disease nowadays and suffering. There is an increasing number of patients, coming to Ayurveda hospitals with the hope of getting cured through Panchakarma therapy, since they could not get completely cured through treatments of modern medical science. Hence Dr. Gopinath has decided to write about this disease first and publish it.

There is a brief description available on this disease in the chapter pertaining to Vatavyadhi in texts like Charaka. With an intention to enlighten in detail on the etiology and treatment of this disease complete information on Pakshaghata (Hemiplegia) from history to treatment including pathya apathya (Congenial/non congenial), divided into different chapters along with his remarks, in an excellent manner has been provided. Everyone will not be able to get a clear insight into this disease by mere reading of texts like Charaka . A clear insight into the disease has been provided by the author, made effortless through diagrams and tables according to the context of the hetu (etiology), samrapti (pathogenesis), lakshana (signs and symptoms) of the disease. Accompanied by an appropriate comparative narration of Hemiplegia and associated conditions of the modern system of medicine, the modern physicians have also been provided with a clear insight to this disease. Pictures on the cover page provide a firsthand perception on the gait of the Pakshaghata (Hemiplegic) patient. The complete shodhana (purificatory) and shamana (palliative) treatment of this disease along with the karmukata (mode of action) of respective kriya (procedures) and yoga (formulations) have also been very well narrated in the chapters pertaining to treatment.

on the whole this is an exemplary work, extremely beneficial as a handbook to medical students, teachers and physicians. I wish Lord Dhanvantari will bestow excellent life, health, wealth and strength to Dr. B. G. Gopinath who intends to write similar texts on a few more diseases under Vatavyadhi.

Mysuru
April 20, 1987

Dr. S. M. Angadi
Principal
Government Ayurveda Medical College
Mysuru

Translator's Note

Professor B.G.Gopinath, an outstanding teacher and a legend among students in the field of Ayurveda, entrusted me with this work of translation of his Kannada volume 'Vatavyadhi' into English more than a decade ago. When his request for translation came, I readily agreed, without realizing the arduous task ahead of me.

Once I started the translation work, I found myself most of the time in a twilight zone. English words conveying the exact meaning of Sanskrit words were simply not there-forget about Ayurveda terms. Very often, when an equivalent term was available, it failed to convey the intended meaning present in the original work.

Professor Gopinath has done commendable work beneficial for students as well as doctors of modern medicine, who are interested in gaining more knowledge pertaining to this difficult disease. The excellent nature of this work was what made me accept this difficult venture.

It is my duty to acknowledge with gratitude the assistance received from Dr. Deepa Kini, currently Professor at Ashwini Ayurveda Medical College, Tumakuru and Dr. Vishal K. Swamy and Dr. Supreeth M.J. then students of postgraduate studies at Sri Kalabhyraveswara Ayurveda

Medical College, Bengaluru. I am also indebted to my daughter Dr. Anupama, who was ever ready in attending to any assistance requested.

I honestly confess that there are shortcomings in this work. I take complete responsibility for these shortcomings, which occurred during translation.

I welcome constructive suggestions.

Bengaluru

August 25, 2023

Dr. M. Ramesh

B.Sc.: M.D (Ayu)

Former Professor

Government Ayurveda Medical College

Bengaluru

CHAPTER – 1

General Discussion on Vatavyadhi

Vatavyadhi has a unique place among the diseases coming under Kaya chikitsa which is an important corollary of Astanga Ayurveda. None of the Ayurveda texts provide separate chapters for the description of nidana (diagnosis) and chikitsa (treatment) of diseases originating from Pitta and Kapha, even though Pitta and Kapha individually and independently can cause diseases. However almost all the textbooks dedicated to Ayurveda reserve one or two chapters exclusively for the nidana (diagnosis) and chikitsa (treatment) of Vatavyadhi. This is a reflection of a special place the study of Vatavyadhi has in Kaya chikitsa. Science of Ayurveda gives special importance to Vatavyadhi compared to diseases of Pitta and Kapha. The reasons for this in the opinion of commentators are as follows.

Reasons for the importance of Vatavyadhi :

1. Vatavyadhis are very powerful diseases.
2. Some of the Vatavyadhis are swift in nature.
3. There are a large number of diseases enumerated under Vatavyadhi.
4. Mostly a cure is difficult to obtain.

5. They require a special line of treatment.
6. Some of the diseases of Vata are critical illnesses.

Vayoho atibalatvena ashukaritvena cha gariyastvat vikaranam dussadhyatvat ashveva atyayakaratvat vishishta chikitsatvat vatavyadhyabhidhanam (Ma.ni.ma.ko.vatavyadhi nidana)

Computation of Vatavyadhi:

An episode as important as this (Vatavyadhi) is equally difficult from the standpoint of academic deliberation. There is no one single disease called Vatavyadhi in the way one deliberates on jwara (fever), swasa (asthma), kasa (cough) etc. This is a signification of a class of several independent extra ordinary diseases caused by Vata. It is only a nomenclature given to a cluster of diseases under the assemblage of Vata roga. Under this appellation specifically nanatmaja disorders of Vata have been described. Here nanatmaja should be construed as that in whose absence the disease will not materialize. Vata nanatmaja carries the meaning that manifestation of the disease is impossible in the absence of Vata, meaning those diseases which appear only in the presence of Vata dushti (vitiated Vata). There is unanimous opinion among all the learned scholars regarding the total number of Vata nanatmaja diseases as 80. However, there is considerable difference of opinion regarding the name, symptoms, etc. of these 80 disorders. A glance through the Vata nanatmaja disorders enumerated in all the pre-eminent texts show that cumulatively the different types of Vata nanatmaja disorders mentioned exceed 80 in number. Thus, one cannot attach too much importance to the number 80 at the present time. The absence of some of the Vatavyadhis or the increased incidence of some others that might have drawn the attention of the respective authors residing in their respective countries at a given period might have led to this type of difference of opinion. There is a school of thought that believes that this difference of opinion occurred because authors of a particular period did not take into account the opinion expressed by erstwhile authors. The contention that even though the authors have reviewed the previous texts during their period in their respective countries, when the diseases mentioned in the previous texts were not seen, such diseases were deleted and those diseases that were newly seen even though they were not mentioned in the previous texts, were included, appears to be more logically appropriate than the contention that the difference of opinion occurred because authors of the later period did not study the texts of the previous period. This narration should not lead the reader to wrongly assume that differences of opinion are dominant in the chapter pertaining to Vatavyadhi. The number of diseases of Vata having differences of opinion are indeed very few in number. A comparative tabulation of this will be given in the second part of the book.

It is an illusion to assume that this episode carries the description of nidana (diagnosis) and chikitsa (treatment) of 80 Vatavyadhis. This episode does not carry the description of nidana panchaka (fivefold diagnosis) and chikitsa (treatment) of all the 80 Vatavyadhis. This is probably because many of the diseases classified as nanatmaja vyadhi are in fact just the signs and symptoms of other disparate diseases and their possibility of being independent diseases being extremely remote. Example: Arasamjnata, Kashayasyata, etc. or else in the absence of any other diseases some abnormalities which incidentally occur are assumed as diseases yet because of fewer symptoms and feeble strength, the description pertaining to their nidana and chikitsa (diagnosis and treatment) might not have been included or there might not have been any new discovery during the stipulated period that can add to the knowledge pertaining to those diseases.

Sushruta samhita does not carry a separate branch of disease called nanatmaja vyadhi. Not only that, many diseases of Vata that are not mentioned in Charaka samhita can be seen in Sushruta samhita, e.g.: Apabahuka.

Apart from this, in Sushruta samhita, 'Apatanaka' has been used as synonymous name for 'Akshepaka' and it considers Apatantraka and Vatarakta as Vatavyadhi. Though in Charaka Samhita indications are available that point towards Vatarakta as Vatavyadhi, a separate chapter has been delineated for the description of this disease. Not only that in Charaka samhita siddhi stana (Chapter 9) Apatanaka and Apatantraka have been mentioned as separate diseases caused due to the vitiation of Hrdaya marma (Heart as vital centre).

According to this samhita this is not a Vatavyadhi.

However, the symptoms of Apatantraka correlate well with the symptoms of Apatantraka as mentioned under Vatavyadhi in Sushruta Samhita. Yet the mention that this vyadhi originates in the Hrdaya (Heart) makes it a difficult context for the reader. Similarly, in Sushruta Samhita Urustambha has been considered and described as a Vatavyadhi. While describing "medavrta vata" in Charaka samhita even though the word "aaddya vata", synonymous name of Urustambha, has been used, the disease Urustambha has been described in a separate chapter.

There are several aspects which require to be pondered in depth in the sphere of treatment pertaining to Vata roga. It is essential to clarify as in which specific disease, the hundreds of tailas, ghritas, guggulu kalpas and rasoushadhis without guggulu that are said to be useful in Vata rogas, are indeed effective.

Which are the medicines to be given when there is dominance of shoola (pain)? It is also essential to clarify as to which is useful when there is karmahani (loss of reflexes) without pain or when the karmavrddhi lakshana (signs and symptoms of exaggerated reflexes) are present. Similarly, what are the medicines to be used when there is Vata prakopa (aggravation of Vata) due to margavarana (occlusion of path)? It is also essential to know the medicines to be given in anomalies arising as a result of dhatu kshaya (depletion of dhatus). On the whole this is sufficient to understand that the episode pertaining to Vatavyadhi is a difficult episode.

The reasons for the difficulty of this episode can be broadly summarized as follows.

1. There is no unanimity of opinion among different acharyas (teachers) regarding the number of *Vatavyadhi.*

2. The indistinct or brief description of *lakshanas (*signs and symptoms*).*

3. Disorderly assignment of some of the anatomical definitions employed during narration of samprapti (pathogenesis) ex: *Sira, snayu, kandara, nadi*.

4. The formidable silence in the matter of roga adhistana (abode of the disease).

5. The intellectual confusion created by the appellation of different nomenclatures to a disease that can be construed as one and the same disease only. Ex: A*kshepa, Ayama, Apatanaka, Apatantraka,* etc.

6. The confusion present with regard to the nomenclature of some of the V*ata rogas*.

   a. ex: *Khalli, Apatantraka* etc.

7. The inability to specify (at times) as to which shamanoushadha (palliative medicine) is superior in which of the specific *Vatavyadhis*.

8. The absence of clear references pertaining to the medicines that are vedana shamaka (palliative) in severe pain.

9. The absence of references pertaining to the medicines that are palliative in severe increase in gati (movements-reflexes) or akshepa (convulsions).

10. The absence of vyavachedaka nidana (differential diagnosis).

11. The non-availability at one and the same locus, medicines that are vyadhi pratyanika (antagonistic to the disease).

Because of the several reasons mentioned above, the chapter pertaining to Vatavyadhi is greatly formidable. Vatavyadhi has to be studied keeping this point in mind. *Vatavyadhis* can be classified for the descriptive purposes as narrated in the ensuing pages.

The classification of *Vatavyadhi* as shown in ensuing pages, in reality, is not narrated upfront by the classics. However, from the standpoint of descriptive felicity, without contradicting the belief of the shastra, an effort is made herein towards classification. The first part of this book by name "*Vatavyadhi*" describes, among the ensuing "7", narrated in the classification, only the disease by name *Pakshaghata, which* is one among the diseases having karma kshaya (diminished power of execution) as its cardinal symptom.

Among the *Vatavyadhis* that have karma *kshaya (*diminished power of execution) as their cardinal symptom, P*akshagata* (Hemiplegia) is an important disease. It will not be wrong to say that among the prominent *Vatavyadhis* *(diseases of Vata)* that come for *Ayurveda* treatment this disease has a mega share. Hence it is necessary to know more about this disease. Keeping this in view, in this first part of the book called Vatavyadhi, all the themes pertaining to Pakshaghata (Hemiplegia) from history to treatment have been described in detail and an effort has been made to show to the students in particular as to how to study a disease from the point of view of Ayurveda.

In common parlance of English language P*akshaghata* is often described as "stroke". The word "stroke" does not always carry the meaning of P*akshaghata*. Conditions such as dysphagia and diplopia can also be called a "stroke". According to Harrison's Textbook of Medicine the disorder stroke sometimes may be a cause, apart from Hemiplegia, also for numbness, sensory deficit, dysphagia, blindness, diplopia, etc. ("A stroke may however give rise to many manifestations other than Hemiplegia, e.g. numbness, sensory deficit, dysphagia, blindness, diplopia, giddiness, and dysarthria"). According to another opinion expressed on stroke in the same text, it is a specific form of aberration appearing acutely and incidentally in a specialized centre of the nervous system. In its severe state the person may suffer from Pakshaghata or may even become unconscious. Such a state is proclaimed by a distinct name called stroke or apoplexy or cerebro vascular accident. (The stroke is a term which connotes the sudden and dramatic development of a focal neurologic deficit. In its severest form, the patient falls hemiplegic and unconscious, an event so striking as to deserve its own separate designation namely apoplexy, stroke or cerebro vascular accident.)

It can be understood from the above substantiation that the word stroke carries a wider meaning than the word P*akshaghata*. *Pakshaghata* as described in *Ayurveda* can be co-related to the modern term Hemiplegia on the basis of the following points.

1. The symptoms of P*akshaghata* resemble the symptoms of Hemiplegia.
2. The literal meaning of the word P*akshaghata* and Hemiplegia are identical.
3. Encyclopedia Britannica describes Hemiplegia as half stroke or paralysis of one side of the body caused by injury to cortico spinal or pyramidal tracts of the central nervous system (En Bri. Vol iv). According to Steadman's Medical Dictionary, “it is a Greek term and means paralysis of one side of the body – loss of power of voluntary movement in a muscle through injury or disease of its nerve supply”. It becomes clear that according to both these texts the word Hemiplegia carries the equivalent meaning to Pakshaghata.

Hemiplegia can be ipsilateral (occurring on the same side as that of brain lesion) or contralateral (occurring on the opposite side to brain lesion) involving muscles of the face and one half of the body (left or right). For accurate treatment, it is important to diagnose whether the patient is having Cerebral stroke (Pakshaghata) or Bell's palsy (Ardita). Bell's palsy is limited to the face because of the involvement of 7th cranial nerve whereas Cerebral ischemia or stroke involves not only lower half of the face but also one half of the body.

Eyes and forehead receive innervation from both hemispheres while lower face only receives innervation from contralateral hemisphere. Lesions that damage the motor cortex such as ischemic strokes, will result in contralateral facial weakness of the lower face only with preservation of muscles of the upper face on both sides, due to dual innervation of the upper face. Patients will have weak smile but will be able to close their eyes tightly and wrinkle the forehead symmetrically. This pattern is the 'central facial weakness', because of the injuries to the Cerebral cortex which is a part of the central nervous system. Lesions that damage the facial nerve (7th cranial) result in ipsilateral (one sided) facial weakness involving both upper and lower face. These lesions are referred as 'peripheral lesions 'because they effect the facial nerve as it exits the brain stem.

Bell's palsy (Ardita) is an acute peripheral facial palsy. There is furrowing of the brows and flattening of the naso labial folds on one side. Strokes involving brain typically cause 'central facial weakness' that involves mouth but spares the eyes and forehead and is very often associated with Hemiplegia or Hemiparesis (weakness on one side)

However rarely, when stroke involves brain stem, there can be weakness of mouth, eyes and forehead.

Drdabala while describing Ardita, in Charaka Samhita, has explained it as

"ardhe tasmin mukhardhe va kevale syat tadarditam"

meaning it is called *Ardita* when deformity is confined to one half of the face or one half of the body with one half of the face. According to Drdabala Ardita can be of two types:

a. *Ardita* – where the deformity is confined to one half of the face (facial paralysis)

b. *Ardita* – deformity of one half of the face + deformity of one half of the body.

This view of Drdabala runs contrary to what one sees in the classical texts of Ayurveda.

From the standpoint of clarity, the term Pakshaghata (Hemiplegia) should comprise of clinical signs and symptoms where in there is deformity of the lower half of the face and / or one half of the body (Ipsilateral or contralateral).

Keeping these points in mind, the Itihasa (History), Hetu (Etiology), Samprapti (Pathogenesis), Lakshana (Signs and symptoms), Sadhyasadhyata (Prognosis), and Chikitsa (Treatment) have been discussed in the ensuing chapters.

Classification of Vatavyadhi

1. Samanya Vatavyadhi

- **Nanatmaja** (Nakhabheda, Anavastita chittatvaadi)
- **Samanyaja** (Vata Jwara, Vataja Atisaradi)

2. Vatavyadhi according to Nidana

- **Janmabala Pravrta** (Pangu, Badhirya, Mookata, Minminatva)
- **Doshabala Pravrta**
  - **Santarpanaja** (due to Margavarana)
    - **Doshavrta**
      - **Mishrita**
      - **Anyonyavrta** — 20
        - 1. Apanavrta Prana
          2. Vyanavrta Prana
          3. Udanavrta Prana
          4. Samanavrta Prana
        - 1. Pranavrta Apana
          2. Vyanavrta Apana
          3. Udanavrta Apana
          4. Samanavrta Apana
        - 1. Udanavrta Samana
          2. Vyanavrta Samana
          3. Apanavrta Samana
          4. Pranavrta Samana
        - 1. Udanavrta Vyana
          2. Samanavrta Vyana
          3. Apanavrta Vyana
          4. Pranavrta Vyana
        - 1. Samanavrta Udana
          2. Vyanavrta Udana
          3. Apanavrta Udana
          4. Pranavrta Udana
      - **Anyadoshavrta** — 10
        - 1. Pittavrta Prana
          2. Kaphavrta Prana
        - 1. Pittavrta Udana
          2 Kaphavrta Udana
        - 1. Pittavrta Vyana
          2. Kaphavrta Vyana
        - 1. Pittavrta Samana
          2. Kaphavrta Samana
        - 1. Pittavrta Apana
          2. Kaphavrta Apana
    - **Dhatvavrta**
      - Rasavrta
      - Raktavrta
      - Mamsavrta
      - Medavrta
      - Astyavrta
      - Majjavrta
      - Shukravrta
    - **Annavrta**
    - **Malavrta**
      - Purishavrta
      - Mutravrta
  - **Apatarpanaja** (due to Dhatukshaya)
- **Sanghatabala Pravrta** (Vrnayama etc)

3. Vatavaishamya bheda

- **Dravyataha**
  - **Vrddhi** (Adhmanadi)
  - **Kshaya**
- **Karmataha**
  - **Vrddhi** (Akshepakadi)
  - **Kshaya** (Pangvadi)
- **Gunataha**
  - **Vrddhi** (Karshya, Parushyadi)
  - **Kshaya** (Vartma-stambhadi)

4. Adhishtana bheda

- **Shareera** (Nakhabhedadi)
- **Manas** (Anavastita chittatvam)
- **Ubhaya** (Apatantraka)

5. Rogamarganusara

- **Bahya rogamargaja**
  - Twakgata
  - Raktagata
  - Mamsagata
  - Medogata
  - Astigata
  - Majjagata
  - Shukragata
- **Abhyantara rogamargaja**
  - Amashayagata
  - Pakvashayagata
  - Gudagata
- **Madhyama rogamargaja**
  - Siragata (Pakshagata, Apabahuka)
  - Snayugata (Ekanga vata, Sarvanga vata)
  - Sandhigata (Sandhivata, Vatakantaka, Kroshtukasheersha, Hanustambha, Manyastambha)
  - Sandhi Marmagata (Apatantraka, Akshepaka, Pakshaghata, Ardita)

6. Samprapti Anusara

- **Dhatu kshayajanya** (Apabahuka, Pakshaghata)
- **Margavaranajanya** (Pakshaghata, Vatarakta, Grdhrasi)

7. Lakshana Anusara

- **Karmakshaya Pradhana** (Pakshaghata, Pangu, Khanja, Mookata)
- **Karmavrddhi Pradhana** (Akshepaka, Kampa)
- **Shula Pradhana** (Grdhrasi, Khalli)

CHAPTER – 2

Beholding The Bygone History

From the time living creatures appeared on this planet earth 'illnesses' have remained a problem. Man has employed and expended all his mental and spiritual powers from time immemorial to prevent or heal these diseases. He has succeeded through relentless and perpetual effort in gaining information pertaining to a number of diseases and discovering their successful treatment to the extent of becoming proud. In this regard it has become a challenge to his abilities, the fact that he is unable to discover the path to successful treatment for a number of other diseases.

All these successes and failures have been systematically enumerated for thousands of years in the medical texts formulated in the respective countries and periods. *Ayurveda* compendiums too join the ranks of many such medical texts. These texts narrate in detail many matters pertaining to the means of preserving the health of a healthy person and curing the illnesses of a diseased person. The successful treatment of many diseases has also been described. *Pakshaghata* (Hemiplegia) is one such disorder where a successful line of treatment has been described.

When one leg and one hand of a person becomes inactivated and useless (symptoms seen in P*akshaghata*) that patient in fact can be assumed to have lost his independence.

He will have to procure every day, the help of others for his daily existential necessities. He will have to depend on them without heeding for likes and dislikes (to help) of such helpful people. Often, he will be incapable of expressing the mental and physical pain he (the patient) is enduring. In such circumstances the tears streaming from his eyes become the only instrument that narrates the history of his sorrow (to the physician). Though P*akshaghata* at all times is not a fatal disease, at the same time it is not an inconsequential, unimportant disease. Also, this is not a new disease. From the description available in the ancient texts like *Charaka Samhita* etc... it can be realized that this is a disorder which is more than 2500 years old. It appears that no other texts except classical texts of *Ayurveda* employed the term *Pakshaghata* or any other synonymous term during the period before 2500 years. *Atharvaveda* which is supposed to be the precursor of *Ayurveda* also does not carry any reference to this disease. The *Sutras*, *Brahmanas*, *Aranyakas* and *Upanishads* which appear at a date subsequent to the *Vedas* also do not provide any information about this disease. Among the available ancient classical texts of India, *Charaka samhita* is the very first text which provides us the information pertaining to the nidana (diagnosis) and c*hikitsa (*treatment*)* of this disease. Even in this text the external etiological factors of *Pakshaghata* have not been separately mentioned. The etiological factors of *Pakshaghata* h a v e to be singled out from the common etiological factors narrated under *Vatavyadhi*. This text carries references to the samprapti (pathogenesis), lakshanas (signs and symptoms), sadyasadhyata (prognosis) and chikitsa sutra (principles of treatment) of this disorder.

However, it does not carry references to any specific shamanoushadha (palliative medicine) that is effective in *Pakshaghata*. Many *Ayurveda* texts of contemporary era appear to have created confusion in the minds of readers by employing *Pakshaghata* and *Ekangavata in synonymous terms*. However, there is no room for such confusion in *Charaka samhita*. There is clear reference here about these two indicating that they are the names of two different diseases. In this context *Charaka chaturanana Chakrapani* has amply elucidated the differences between these two. It can be said that A*charya Agnivesha* has pinpointed towards the moola *adhishtana (*original abode*)* (*Shiro Marma*) of *Pakshaghata* by describing c*heshta* nasha *(*loss of movements*) and other* symptoms while explaining the *lakshanas (*signs and symptoms*)* of Shiro *marmabhighata (*trauma to vital centre, head*)* in the *Trimarmiya adhyaya* of siddhistana.

Among the 80 Vata rogas mentioned in this *Samhita, Pakshaghata* is also one.

Sushruta samhita also recognizes this disease as one among *Maha Vata rogas*. This s*amhita* also mentions *samprapti (*pathogenesis*)*, *lakshanas (*signs and symptoms) *sadhyasadhyata (*prognosis*)* as well as the *chikitsa sutras (*principles of treatment*)* of *Pakshaghata*. The highlighting of localized treatments *Mastishkya*, *Shirobasti,* which have not been directly mentioned while explaining the treatment of *Pakshaghata* in *Charaka samhita,* authenticates the belief that the moola *adhistana (*core abode*)* of *Pakshaghata* as *Mastishka (Brain)* existed even during those times. There is one feature which cannot be seen in any of the available s*amhita granta*, but is seen in this s*amhita,* i.e., the minimum total duration in the treatment of *Pakshghata*. It is said that continuous treatment for a minimum of 3 – 4 months should be given.

Uniqueness seen in this s*amhita* is the clear-cut direction as to which specific *taila (*oil*)* has to be used in P*akshaghata* for what specific purpose - a*bhyanga (unction), nasya (*nasal instillation) etc. Treatment of P*akshaghata* mentioned in this text is comparatively more extensive than that mentioned in C*haraka samhita.* If taken in that view one can see a number of different *yogas (*formulations*)* taila (oils) etc. that can be employed in *Pakshaghata,* in the texts that belong to the contemporary period of *Sushruta samhita* but it can be said that they do not describe the chikitsa sutra (principles of treatment) as extensively as in S*ushruta samhita.*

Ashtanga sangraha and *Ashtanga hrdaya* though describe the n*idana (*diagnosis*) and chikitsa (*treatment*)* of P*akshaghata* (A.hr.Ni. 15/38 – 39 and A.hr. Chi 21 -24), no specific contribution on this subject can be seen. The role of these two texts in perpetuating systematically the light of knowledge pertaining to this disease extant so far and handing it over to the next generation should be kept in our perspective.

Kashyapa samhita also mentions "P*akshavadha"as* one among 80 *Vatavyadhis (*diseases of Vata*)*. However, description pertaining to its nidana (diagnosis) and mode of *chikitsa (*treatment*)* is not accessible (Ka. S. Su 27/28).

Bhela samhita do not make any reference to *Pakshavadha.* However, in the episode pertaining to treatment of Vatavyadhi it has been mentioned that *Paksha graha* is one among the 80 V*ata rogas*. It is a contentious subject as to whether by the word P*akshagraha* one should recognize P*akshavadha* or whether it is a totally different V*ata vikara.*

Harita samhita makes reference to P*akshaghata* along with E*kangavata* (Chapter 3, 20/28). It has been merely mentioned here that P*akshaghata* is a difficult to cure disease where *Vataghna chikitsa (*treatment for elimination of vata*)* should be employed. Other than this there are no other special points mentioned.

Madhava nidana mentions exclusively the nidanatmaka (etiological) aspects of P*akshaghata* whereas C*hakradutta* explains only those aspects that pertains to *chikitsa (*treatment*)*. Since the subject matter of these two texts being *nidanatmaka (*etiological*)* and *chikitsatmaka (therapeutical)* respectively, it is only apt that subject matter pertaining to roga nidana (etiology of disease) has been mentioned in *Madhava nidana* and subject matter pertaining to *chikitsa (*treatment*)* has been mentioned in C*hakradutta.* We can see in C*hakradutta* the kwata (decoctions), *kalka (pulp)* and taila *kalpanas (*formulations *of* oils*)* that are useful for *nasya (*nasal instillation*), basti (medicated enema)* and other treatment forms employed in *Pakshaghata*. In this text phrases "P*akshavata*" (Ch.Da.22/27), *Pakshaghata* and

Ardhanga shosha have been employed synonymously (Ch. Da.22/23).

Sharangdhara samhita being a text that deals with topics related to *Bhaishajya kalpana (*medicinal formulations) any kind of description pertaining to *nidana (diagnosis)* and *chikitsa (*treatment*)* of P*akshaghata* is not accessible here. However, the word P*akshaghata* has been mentioned while narrating the qualities of M*aha Manjishtadi kwata* and M*ashadi nasya* (Sha.Ut.8/36 – 37). Probably this is the only text which prescribes M*aha Manjishtadi kwata* (*Madhyama khanda*2/137 – 142) in P*akshaghata*. This is a special feature of this text.

The general line of treatment of *Pakshaghata* has been narrated in K*alyanakaraka* of *Ugradityacharya* where it is mentioned that P*akshaghata* with *sparsha hani (*numbness*)* or vedana (pain) and angashosha (emaciation of bodily parts) is impossible to cure.

Among the texts of the Middle Ages it appears that the text *Vangasena*, verbatim repeats nidanatmaka vishaya (etiological aspects) of *Pakshaghata* mentioned in *Sushruta samhita*. Kwata (decoction), churna (pulverized powder) or vati (pills) and taila kalpanas (formulations of oil) can be seen in this text in relation to treatment. Most of the yogas (formulations) seen here are repetitions of the yogas (formulations) mentioned in *Chakradutta*. It has been said about *Pakshaghata* that puranatva (chronicity) of the disease is an indicator of incurability. The word "Pakshavata" has also been employed here as a simile for Pakshaghata.

Pakshaghata, Ardhangavata, Ekangavata etc. have been referred while explaining Vatavyadhi in *Basavarajeeya*. It is a specialty of this book that Ardhangavata has been mentioned as if it is the name of a different disease, without using it as a synonymous word for Pakshaghata. It can be seen in this text also that the puranatva (chronicity) of the disease is an indicator of the incurability of Pakshaghata. It is a specialty of this text that while narrating the lakshanas (signs and symptoms) of Pakshaghata it mentions lakshanas (signs and symptoms) totally different from the narration in classical texts of antecedent period. This text narrates that shoola (pain) kampa (tremor), etc... aapaadatala mastaka (from sole of the feet to the vertex) in one half of the body is a symptom of Pakshaghata.

These symptoms of Pakshaghata appear somewhat incredulous when compared to other classical texts. It is reminiscent here that the above two symptoms have not been mentioned as salient features in other classical texts. Similarly, a Vata roga by name Parshwavata has also been narrated. Not only that the symptoms of Parshwavata and Ardhangavata have been discussed separately and it has been pointed out that they are different from Pakshaghata (their symptoms do not correlate to Pakshaghata). In adducing Pakshaghata as a very tenacious Vatavyadhi and prescribing Agni chikitsa – agni karma (Branding) for it, from the standpoint of treatment, this book is a first-rate testifier of a new step forward. According to this text, 'Kalakantaka rasa "is a divine medicine for Pakshaghata.

Yogaratnakara also mentioned Pakshaghata as one among 80 Vatavyadhi. Maharasnadi kwata, Mahalaxminarayana taila, Dwa trimshatika guggulu, Laghu vishagarbha taila, Vatarakshasa – these are the manifold medicines mentioned for Pakshaghata. *Bhavaprakasha* also carries a description of Pakshaghata. Many of the medicines mentioned in *Yogaratnakara* are not seen here. It can be said that references pertaining to vishishta yogas (specialized formulations) for Pakshaghata are few in this text. There is reference to Pakshaghata in the three yogas – Trayodashanga guggulu, Madhyama narayana taila and Maha saindhavadhya taila.

The chikitsa sutras (principles of treatment) of Pakshaghata have been narrated in *Rasaratnakara*. Some useful yogas (formulations) have also been mentioned. "Ardhangavatari rasa"is one among them.

"Ardhavapurvata" has been used as a synonymous word for the Pakshaghata in the thirteenth century work *Rasendra Chintamani.* This name is a new addition to the group of synonymous words for Pakshaghata that were in vogue till this date. " Pindi rasa" is said to be a divine medicine for Pakshaghata.

Rasendrasara sangraha not only advocates the use of "Vatagajankusha rasa" in Pakshaghata but also employs the word "Ardhavapurvata" as synonymous for Pakshaghata.

Rasa tarangini advocates the use of Vishatinduka in Pakshaghata. It also contraindicates its use in certain exceptional situations. This theme is not to be seen in any of the texts till date.

The prescription of Avagaha sweda (immersed diaphoresis) in Taila droni (a tub filled with oil) (Va.Vya.31) or Kanjika droni (tub of fermented gruel) is a unique contribution of Bhaishajyaratnavali which carries an excellent compilation of many kalpanas (formulations) mentioned in ancient texts. It is a matter of contemplation here that this treatment for Pakshaghata has not been mentioned in any other text. Pana (oral administration), Basti (enema), Abhyanga (unction), Karnapurana (instillation to ears), Akshitarpana (ocular nourishment), Tailadroni avagahana (Immersed diaphoresis in oil filled tub) are mentioned as lines of treatment in Pakshaghata. The ambit of lines of treatment explained in this book is considerably more than in many other classical texts. The author has employed the term "Pakshavata" in place of "Pakshaghata". Among the yogas (formulations) narrated here Yogendra rasa, Rasaraja rasa, Nakuladya ghrita are worth mentioning Other yogas (formulations) are mere repetitions of what is mentioned in the previous texts.

Dr. Ashananda Pancharatna, in the first part of his book "*Vyadhi Vignana*" has compared Pakshaghata to Hemiplegia of modern medical science and has enumerated the lakshanas (signs and symptoms) of Hemiplegia mentioned in modern medicine as symptoms of Pakshaghata. Continuing with his explanations he has written the differential diagnosis on the basis of internal causes such as embolism and internal hemorrhage. He has also discussed how to carry out its treatment both from the standpoint of the Modern system as well as Ayurveda.

Dr. Sudarshana Shastry in the *Vidyotini Hindi teeka* (commentary) of Madhava nidana has correlated Pakshaghata to Hemiplegia in a competent manner. He has also explained in broad terms the Mastishka vikrta rupi samprapti (Cerebral pathogenesis) occurring in Pakshaghata.

Vaidya Haridasa panchanana in his book has described briefly Pakshaghata based on Ayurveda, Unani, and Modern systems of medicine. One can say that this book does not make any contribution so far as the topic of nidana (etiology) of this disease is concerned. Some of the sentences written by this author makes one feel that he has wrongly cognized Ardhangavata (Paraplegia) as Pakshaghata. He mentions that change in colour on the vikrta parshwa (aberrant side) is an indicator of incurability of disease and absence of change in colour is an indicator of curability and opines that the origin of this concept is from Unani. This is not seen in Ayurveda. The author has described treatment of Pakshaghata at two different places. The attributes of the line of the treatment he has given, at once, neither belongs to Ayurveda nor to the Modern system of medicine. The classical assumptions in this regard have been discarded either through ignorance or through negligence by his advocacy of calomel for virechana (laxation) and by the assertion that glycerin enema is superior to virechana (laxation). At another place continuing with the treatment of Pakshaghata the use of Mashadi kwata and Mashadi taila have been narrated. Apart from these some yogas (formulations) from one's own experience have also been mentioned. He has praised as very effective Swacchanda bhairava rasa and exclusive use of Kajjali in Pakshaghata.

The greatest compilatory text pertaining to Rasa shastra belonging to the twentieth century *Rasayogasagara* do not provide anything special pertaining to Pakshaghata other than some formulations- Indravaruni rasa, Pakshaghata vidhwamsana rasa, Ekangaveera rasa etc. This text also employs a synonymous word called "Pakshavata". Describing the use of Pakshaghata vidhwamsana rasa it narrates distinctively as to at what dose, the number of times per day, with what anupana (ensuing potion) and for how many days this should be given. This is a special feature rarely seen generally in ancient classical texts. The complete description of dose, duration, anupana, total duration of medication pertaining to a yoga (classical formulation) is very rare in most of the texts. The honour of narrating all these points in each yoga (formulation) should go to the author.

What are the classical preparations more beneficial at what stages of Pakshaghata – nutana, jeerna and upadamshajanya (acute, chronic and syphilitic) has been written on the basis of long experience by Swami Krishnanandji in his *Rasatantrasara or Siddhaprayoga Sangraha* (Hindi). A compendium has been provided in the last pages of the book to enable one to search as to which medicine is to be given at what stage. It becomes very easy for the physician to decide the employment of shamanoushadha (palliative treatment) in Pakshaghata on this basis.

The information pertaining to nidana (diagnosis) and chikitsa (treatment) of Pakshaghata as provided in classical texts from antiquity to important Ayurveda books of the twentieth century has so far been gained. A broad acquaintance pertaining to the developments that have occurred or ensuing regarding this disease from the middle of the twentieth century onwards can be reckoned henceforth.

The exclusive use of Mashadi taila in Pakshaghata has been employed by Dr. R.H Anand and Dr. M.H.K. Mehta. According to one of their reports (Ayu October 1975) it is observed that the upper extremity of vikrta parshwa (deformed half) healed more rapidly than the lower extremity. Some scholars have experimented exclusively with Shiro basti (cumulative medicament on the head). According to them this helps specially in reducing the abnormalities of joint movement, sleep and speech as also in assisting improvement of locomotor efficacy (Ayu, July 1975). Some other scholars have employed virechana (laxation) and snehadhara sveda (oleaginous cascade diaphoresis) in Pakshghata and have reported them to be highly efficacious. Thus, research has been conducted and is still being carried on by several scholars in different parts of the country. It is regretted that this small volume cannot carry all these descriptions.

Even after perceiving foremost texts pertaining to roga nidana (diagnosis of disease) and chikitsa (treatment) ranging from *Charaka samhita* up to the twentieth century and a broad glimpse of research related to study of treatment of Pakshaghata, dimensions of its history will not be complete unless reference is made here to another important aspect of this disease. Therefore, it appears pertinent to add a few words pertaining to traditional treatments based on experience, which can be regarded as another dimension of the history of this disease.

There are a number of traditional physicians in different

parts of the country. They do not have profound knowledge of Ayurveda to any great extent. (Exceptionally there are some with profound knowledge of Ayurveda gained through self-study). Even then there are also some who gained experience by staying with elders in the family who were giving medicines for some of the illnesses and based on such foundation, there are some who diagnosed those diseases and provided identical treatment. There are a number of physicians in this group who use the term "Lakwa" or "Parshwa Vayu" for Pakshaghata and provide treatment for the same. There are a number of patients who have recovered with this kind of treatment. Meaning the treatment given by such people can also be successful is proven by experience. Their treatment may not be purely classical. However, from the standpoint of financial, commercial and time factor this should be pondered over here as a simple and easy treatment. Even today there are such traditional physicians in Karnataka who provide simple and easy treatments. There is sufficient scope for impartial research by educated qualified physicians on the treatment given by such physicians. One such instance is the already reported Ankola chikitsa – agni chikitsa for "Lakwa" carried out by Udupi Ayurveda College and found useful. This is worthy of emulation.

CHAPTER – 3

Paribhasha – Paryaya Nama Prakarana
Treatise on Definition – Synonyms

Definition of Pakshaghata

This is one among the 80 avishkrtatama (differentially well-known and understood) nanatmaja (originating from solitary dosha) vyadhi (disease) of Vata dosha. This is a difficult to treat disease with classical symptoms of loss of function in the left hand and left leg or right hand and right leg of the body. This is known by the name "Lakwa" or "Parshvavayu".

1. "Hatvaikam marutaha paksham dakshinam vamameva va "(Cha. Chi.28/23)

2. "Vamam dakshinam va paksham hanti "(Aruna Dutta)

Synonyms and Their Description

The following words have been used to mean Pakshaghata in diverse Ayurveda texts.

1. Pakshaghata	**2. Pakshavadha**
3. Pakshavata	**4. Ardhangavata**
5. Ardhavapurvata	**6. Ardhangashosha**
7. Pakshagraha	**8. Ardhangaghata**
9. Ekanga vata	

Since it helps to understand the different dimensions of the disease by precise appraisal of the origin and the description of the meaning of the above said words, the descriptive derivation of each word is given below to the extent possible.

1. **Pakshaghata:** Of all synonyms for this disease this is the single most commonly used word in almost all the classical texts. This is a compound word made of two different words. This contains two words "paksha" and "aghata". Among these two the first word paksha carries many meanings in Sanskrit language. For example:

a. Krishna paksha, Shukla paksha employed during the perusal of time span "kala". Here the word paksha has been used to denote a period of 15 days.

"Pakshaha panchadasha ahoratraha/
Sacha dvividaha shukla pakshaha, krishna paksho apara samjnehe// (sha.ka.dhru)

b. *"pakshachedodyatam shakram"* In the present context of "Indra has set out for pakshachheda", the word paksha has been used to mean a "specialized structure of birds" – the wings. (pakshinaam *avayava visheshaha - ra* 4-40)

c. The words poorva paksha - utthara paksha have been used in the context of pratipadana (espousal) during the course of vada (polemics). In this context the word paksha is used to mean the presentation of contrary opinions. {... virodhe - Shabda kalpa druma).

d. Another meaning for this word carries the connotation of left or right side of the body (...bahu parshva uru janghadi bhagan). The word paksha in Pakshaghata is used with this meaning. Though a part of the body can be divided into upper (urdhwa) and lower part (adho bhaga / paksha) in the present context the commentators have clarified that from the word paksha, the right and left half should be discerned. This clarification has been given through the examples of *ardhanareeshwaravat natu nrsimhavat.* Meaning the manner in which we apprehend the right and left parts of the body through the word *ardha nareeshwara* similarly in Pakshaghata the left and right side should be comprehended and have been told not to cognise *urdhwa and adho bhaga* (upper and lower part) as in "nrsimha". Even in the core texts, it has been clearly mentioned as "*vamam dakshinam va paksha*". From this it becomes clear that Pakshaghata always comes into manifestation either on the left or right side (of the body).

The second word "aghata" of "Pakshaghata" indicates as to what happens to the right or left side of the body. The word aghata originates from anj prathyaya poorvaka "han" dhatu. Ghata carries the meaning "to destroy". Meaning, even though the literal meaning indicates the destruction of the part affected by the disease, in the present context it is reasonable to assume merely the obvious meaning of functional deficiency of the part. More details in this regard will be given in the appropriate ensuing context.

This compound word has been especially employed in the following texts.

1. Charaka samhita	2. Sushruta samhita
3. Ashtanga sangraha	4. Ashtanga hrdaya
5. Sharangadhara samhita	6. Chakradutta
7. Yogaratnakara	8. Harita samhita
9. Vangasena	10. Bhavaprakasha
11. Bhaishajyaratnavali	12. Kalyanakaraka
13. Rasayogasagara	14. Rasendrasara sangraha
15. Rasatarangini, etc.	

2. **Pakshavadha:** This is also a compound word. The word Paksha here carries the same meaning as described earlier. The word "Vadha" originates from han+anj "han" moola *dhatu* (verb root). Its meaning 'prana viyoga phalaka vyapara' (a venture plank leading to uncoupling of life force) meaning an act that endangers life. However, the word vadha in Pakshavadha should be understood only as functional deficiency of one hand and one leg of left or right side of the body (pranahani kriye) and should not be construed that danger to life itself (pranahani) is the cardinal symptom in Pakshavadha.This word is wholly synonymous to the word Pakshaghata.

Both the words mentioned above are words that indicate the vyakti stana (realm of manifestation) and the cardinal lakshana (symptom) of the disease. The word Pakshavadha can be mainly seen in the texts of Kashyapa Samhita and Vangasena.

3. **Pakshavata:** This compound word also carries two words Paksha + Vata. Among these, meaning of the first word "*paksha*" has already been stated. The second word "vata" is one among the *tridoshas* in Ayurveda. It originates from the dhatu (verb root) "va" carrying the meaning of "*gati*", "*gandhana*". *'Va gati gandhanayoho'.* Gati means movement, gandhana means indication or cognition of knowledge. This word indicates that the disease Pakshavata is caused by vata dosha which can cause aberrations related to *kriya* (motor) and *samjna* (sensory) functions. This compound word points towards a dosha that is a part of *samprapti ghataka* (component of pathogenesis) as well as *vyakti stana* (realm of manifestation). This word is mainly seen in Vangasena.

4. **Ardhangavata:** From the historical perspective this is an *arvacheena shabdha* (proximate word). This word is found to have been employed in Rasaratnakara and Rasatarangini. This is a compound word formed of three words ardha + anga + vata. Here the word "*anga*" is used to carry the equivalent meaning of "*shareera*" (body) and "ardha" to carry the equivalent meaning of "paksha" (half). It indicates that in this disease there is an aberration in half of the body and vata is existent in this disease as cardinal *samprapti ghataka* (component of pathogenesis).

5. **Ardhavapurvata:** This is a compound word comprising of three words ardha + vapuhu + vata. It is said that here vapuhu means *"upyante dehantara bhoga sadhana bheeji bhutani karmani iti vapuhu"* (Sha. ka. dru). The place where the deeds of past life which is the cause for happiness

and sorrow in this life comes into manifestation is called vapuhu. This is a synonymous word for the word shareera. This word is equivalent to ardhanga vata mentioned earlier. This word can be specifically seen in Rasaratna samucchaya and Rasachandamshu.

6. **Ardhangashosha:** This is also a compound word formed of three words ardha + anga + shosha. The first two words carry the same meaning mentioned earlier (4 and 5). The word shosha is distinctive here. Shosha means desiccation or emaciation (*shushyatyanena iti shoshaha*). In reality among patients of Pakshaghata sometimes because of disuse of structures involved in aghata (aberration) it is found that the structure becomes emaciated in the course of time (atrophy due to disuse). Hence the word ardhanga shosha might have been employed. Apart from that, while explaining samprapti (pathogenesis) of this disease having said "*sira snayurvishoshyacha*", emaciation of the snayu (muscles) has been indicated. From this standpoint also this synonymous word is apt. This is a paryaya nama (synonymous name) indicative of vyaktistana (realm of manifestation), samprapti (pathogenesis) and lakshana (signs and symptoms).

Charakachaturanana Chakrapani has employed this word in his therapeutic text 'Chakradutta'. One can behold his use of word "ardhangagata vata" carrying equivalent meaning to the word "ardhanga vata" as synonymous.

7. **Pakshagraha:** This word has been cited in Bhela samhita while expounding Vata vikaras. The word paksha here carries the same meaning as explained earlier. The

meaning of "graha" is to grasp - (*ga-ei-grahani*-(S*ha. ka.dru*); grasping *grahayati-grahat*i-(Sha.ka.dru). Perhaps in Pakshaghata the word graha may have been employed to indicate the restricted movements seen in the shakha (limbs). Sometimes in Pakshaghata there will not be complete loss of movement of the vikrta shakha (aberrant limbs). The word Pakshagraha can be employed when such incomplete loss of movement occurs. This synonymous word is indicative of the vyakti stana (realm of manifestation) as well as lakshanas (signs and symptoms). The word Parshwagraha is also used at many places in the shastra (classics). The word parshwa has been sometimes used as synonymous for the word paksha. Hence it is natural to vacillate as to whether parshwagraha can be considered as a synonymous name for pakshagraha. However, when the technical contexts of the employment of the word parshwagraha is perceived, it is clear that it cannot be a synonymous name for pakshagraha. It becomes apparent that parshwagraha is a disparate symptom.

8. **Ardhangaghata:** Even though there are several synonyms in the classical texts, some modern Ayurveda scholars of the twentieth century have brought into vogue a word called "Ardhangaghata". The word ardhanga has been employed instead of the word paksha in Pakshaghata. This too is an indicator of the vyakti stana (realm of manifestation) and lakshanas (symptoms).

9. **Ekangavata:** Herein there are three words eka+anga+vata. Ekanga carries the meaning of one avayava (limb). Meaning a word that can be employed when one leg or one hand alone becomes vikrta (aberrant). This word

has been used as synonyms for Pakshaghata by Vagbhata and Madhava. However, the word ekanga do not carry the meaning of one paksha (half) at all. Pakshaghata do not always happen to one hand or one leg alone (it happens always to one hand and one leg). Therefore, it does not appear appropriate to employ the word Ekangavata for Pakshaghata. Chakrapani, the commentator of Charaka has clarified that Ekangavata and Pakshaghata are two separate entities. Dalhana has clearly stated that "ekasminnangeya *utpadhyate sa ekanga vikaraha" (su.sutra 14/30).*

A theme common to all the synonymous names described earlier is the employment of one or the other word depicting the vyakti stana (realm of manifestation) of the disease and its lakshana (symptoms). Highlighting the vikrti (aberration) to one paksha (half) is very common (in all the synonyms except the word "Ekangavata"). Some of the words among them are indicative of samprapti (pathogenesis) and lakshana (symptoms). Some are indicative of the dominant doshas causative of the disease. They are shown in the following table.

Indicator of vyakti stana (Realm of manifestation) samprapti, (pathogenesis) Lakshana (symptoms)	**Indicator of vyakti stana (Realm of manifestation) and dosha**	**Indicator of vyakti stana (Realm of manifestation) and lakshana (symptoms)**
1. Pakshavadha 2. Ardhangashosha 3. Ardhangaghata 4. Pakshaghata	1. Ardhangavata 2. Ardhavapurvata 3. Pakshavata 4. Ardhangagatavata	1. Pakshagraha

CHAPTER – 4

Hetu Prakarana

Treatise on Etiology

Every karya (effect) has a karana (cause). Pakshaghata is a karya (effect). Even for that, one or the other karana (cause) has to be present. Specific causes for this disease have not been mentioned in the classical texts. This possibly carries the meaning that till the time of creation of these texts no specific cause could be found. Hence samanya nidana (common etiological factors) alone have been narrated for Vata rogas. To say that all the common etiological factors of Vata roga should cause all the Vatavyadhis and all those causative factors of Vata causes Pakshaghata, is only a polemic and cannot be realistic. Even though Ashtanga hrdaya nidana Chapter 16, Sushruta nidana chap.1 as well as other contexts narrate the types of vikaras (abnormalities) caused by each of the five Vatas and A.h. ni.ch.16 narrates the prakopaka karana (aggravating factors) for these, we are yet to reach a position to say specifically as to which of the Vatavyadhis are caused by which of the specific causative factors of Vata vitiating which of the specific denomination of Vata dosha. All the direct and indirect causative factors mentioned for Pakshaghata and Vata prakopa (aggravation) in Ayurveda, in different contexts, when compiled and pondered over, it becomes clear that the internal causative factors for Hemiplegia narrated in the Modern systems can be the causative factors for Pakshaghata from the standpoint of Ayurveda also. Generally, Pakshaghata may be caused by margavarana (occlusion of the path), asrk srava (hemorrhage), shirobhighata (traumas to the head). Apart from that since some of the symptoms of this disease are seen in marmaghata of Kakshadhara marma (trauma to vital center at anterio inferior axillary line involving brachial plexus) and Lohitaksha marma (vital centre involving the dorsal and ventral aspects of axillary joint), these also have been deliberated only to the extent necessary in this chapter.

1. **Margavarana (Occlusion of the Conduit): -** Internal causative factors for Vata prakopa (aggravation of Vata) are two, margavarana (Occlusion of the conduit) is one among them.

vayordhatukshayat kopaha margasyavaranena (Cha. chi 28/42).

Margavarana means obstruction to the path of flow of dosha dhatu and mala. Formation of blood clots (thrombosis) in the blood vessels that supply to the brain, air embolism, arbuda (tumors) or vidradi (abscess), etc. create obstruction to the blood circulation to the Mastishka (Brain). Because of this Pakshaghata (Hemiplegia) may occur due to deficiency in the act of nourishment through rasa and rakta (nutrient plasma and blood) to the unique organ brain (ischemic brain). Even though our acharyas (teachers) have not mentioned anywhere tumours etc. as causative of Pakshaghata but since they have mentioned that Vata prakopa (aggravation of Vata) occurs through margavarana (occlusion of conduit), it will not be wrong on our part to understand that they cause Pakshaghata through aggravation of Vata by causation of margavarana (occlusion to the conduit).

2. **Asrk sravana (Bloodletting):** - In fact this carries the meaning of bloodletting. However, from the standpoint of outcome, blood flowing out on its own or bloodletting both are identical. Therefore, the outcome of the bleeding has to be cognized, irrespective of active or passive blood flow. This kind of bleeding occurring in the region of the brain can cause Pakshaghata.

1. Atyushne...Ajnairvidham...Atipravartate tadatipravartam... pakshaghatam ekangavikaramcha (Su.suthra 14/30)

2. Garbhini sootika ....asrk srute pakshaghatam .... (Ma.ni)

In the above reference it has been indicated that in reality Pakshaghata can occur as a result of Vata prakopa (aggravation of Vata) due to dhatu kshaya (depletion of supportive elements) resulting from excessive outflow of blood. It stands to common logic that Pakshaghata may also result because of margavaranajanya Vata prakopa (aggravation of Vata arising due to obstruction of the conduit), if bleeding occurring in the brain do not flow out, forming a clot 'in situ'. Hence asrk sravana (hemorrhage) has also been considered as one of the causative factors herein. This kind of abhyantara rakta srava (internal hemorrhage) is seen in pravrdha raktachapa (hypertension), subdural hemorrhage and dhamani katinyata (atherosclerotic changes) etc.

3. **Shirobhighata (Trauma to the Head):** - Drdabalacharya while narrating the consequences of shiro

marmabhighata (trauma to the head) in Trimarmeeya adhyaya of Charaka samhita siddhi stana states "*shirasyabhihate manyastambardita ....cheshtanasha ....vadana jihwadeeni*". In this context most of the abnormalities narrated as likely to occur because of shiro marmabhighata (trauma to the vital center of head), are Vata vikara (abnormality of Vata). Among them an abnormality called "*chestanashaha*" (loss of function) is one. This is a specialized feature seen in Pakshaghata (akarmanyo *vichetanaha*). There is a possibility of internal hemorrhage in shiro marmabhighata (trauma to the head). This can also cause Pakshaghata. Traumas need not necessarily be exclusively external. The reference in sutra stana of Charaka samhita "indriyani *samashritya* ... *yada malaha upaghatopatapabhyam te* " is a hint to the fact that trauma can also be the result of abhyantara (internal) dosha. The mention in this verse that aggravated doshas cause upaghata (morbidity) and upatapa (distress) is a signification of trauma due to dosha. This kind of abhighata (trauma) due to dosha can result in Pakshaghata through mastishka shota (cerebral edema) or mastishkagata rakta srava (cerebral hemorrhage). Mutra vishamayata (toxicity due to renal failure), dhamani khatinyata (atherosclerosis) are examples of trauma due to doshas (dosha abhighata).

4. **Marmabhighata (Trauma to Vital Centre): -** It is not appropriate to say that trauma to any one of the 107 marmas (vital centres) causes Pakshaghata. It is indicated that if trauma occurs to Lohitaksha (vital centre at the root of the limbs) and Kakshadhara (vital centre in the axilla) there is a possibility of occurrence of Pakshaghata .

"tatra lohitakshayenna maranam pakshaghato va"
" *kakshadhare pakshaghatam "(* su.sha 6/24)

Lohitaksha marma is a sira marma (vascular vital center) located at the urumoola (root of thighs). Kakshadhara is a snayu marma (muscular vital part) located between the vakshas (chest) and kaksha (axilla).

Dr.Ramaraksha Pathak has opined that Lohitaksha marma comprises

a) Femoral triangle and structures therein

b) The third part of axillary blood vessels along with branches of brachial plexus and proximal part of brachial vessels. He observes that Kakshadhara marma is the "first and second part of axillary vessels and brachial plexus".

It is a challenging invitation to future research scholars to prove the fact that trauma to these two vital centres causes Pakshaghata. At present nothing more can be said about this.

5. **Vidradi (Abscess) :- It** has been said that when doshas become (occluded), if occlusion is derelicted and not dislodged upadrava (supervenient afflictions) such as Vidradhi (abscess) etc can occur.

Vidradhi pleeha hrdroga gulma....
Bhavantyupadravastesham avrtanam upekshanat/ (A.hr.Ni 19/58)

Because of margavarana (occlusion of conduits), meaning if any kind of obstruction takes place in the specified blood vessels of the brain, a Vidradhi (abscess) develops in that region in course of time, aggravating margavarana (occlusion of conduits) and may cause Pakshaghata. An effort has been made to elucidate this topic in the context of samprapti (pathogenesis) of Pakshaghata.

The onset of Pakshaghata may be at a sheegra gati (rapid pace) or manda gati (slow pace). Varied nidana (etiology) (abhyantara nidana - internal etiology) is said to be responsible for these two forms of onset. Based on these, causative factors can be classified as sheegrotpadaka (rapid onset) and mandotpadaka (slow onset).

This has been shown in a tabular format below.

HETU (ETIOLOGY)

Sheegrotpadaka (Rapid Onset)	**Mandotpadaka (Slow Onset)**
1. Mastishkagata raktasrava (Cerebral hemorrhage) due to raktachapa (hypertension) or dhamanikatinya (atherosclerosis)	1. Mastishkarbuda (Brain tumour)
2. Embolism	2. Mastishka vidradhi
3. Thrombosis	3. Sub-acute meningitis
4. Uremia (Mutra vishamayata), etc.	4. Subdural hemorrhage
	5. Raktadhatukshayajanya Vata prakopa, etc. (Aggravated Vata due to depletion of blood)

Among those narrated above Arbuda (Tumors), Vidradi (Abscess) Embolism, Thrombosis, Mastishkagata raktasrava (cerebral haemorrhage), etc are deemed as margavarodhaka karana(obstructive etiology) and the remaining can be understood as marmabhighataka karana (etiological factors causing trauma to the marmas) due to doshas.

Nidanartakara roga (Secondary diseases originating from primary disease) :- Pravrdha Raktachapa (Hypertension), Upadhamsha (Syphilis), Dhamanikatinyata (Atherosclerosis), Mastishkagata vidradhi (Cerebral abscess), Mutra vishamayata (Uremia), Mastiskagata raktavahini kshata (injury to cerebral blood vessel), Mastishkavarana shota (Meningitis), etc.

Margavarodhaka nidana (Obstructive etiology):-Vega sandharana (Inhibition of natural urges), Ama (incompletely formed toxic nutrient element due to unaccomplished digestion), Marmabhighata (trauma to vital centres), etc.

Dhatukshayakaraka nidana (Consumptive etiology):- Vyavaya (Coitus), Ratri jagarana (Wakefulness at night), Consumption of ruksha (rough), laghu (light), alpa ahara (meagre food), Raktamokshana (Phlebotomy), Vyayama (Exercise), Shoka (Sorrow), Chinta (Worries) Rogakarshana (Emaciation due to diseases), Sheegra yana (Swift journey) Langhana (Starvation).

CHAPTER - 5

Samprapti Prakarana
Treatise on Pathogenesis

It will be difficult to understand with clarity the samprapti (pathogenesis) of many of the diseases mentioned in the shastras (classical texts) if verses related to the samprapti (pathogenesis) of the disease narrated in the relevant context alone is considered. This applies also to Pakshaghata. An accurate lucid perception of its samprapti (pathogenesis) cannot be gained just by reading only one or two verses describing the samprapti (pathogenesis) of Pakshaghata. It will not become clear as to in which part of the body the source of vikrti (abnormality) in Pakshaghata lies. We will have to compile and describe the innumerable themes narrated at different places for a proper understanding. Therefore, an effort is made here- in to explain samprapti (pathogenesis) by bringing to one place, many themes essential to understand samprapti (pathogenesis) narrated at different places. It becomes helpful from the standpoint of treatment of whatever disease if samprapti (pathogenesis) of that disease is studied through samprapti ghataka (components of pathogenesis). Samprapti ghataka (components of pathogenesis) are not new concepts. Dr. K.Sadashiva Sharma has compiled this topic and systematized it in his book *Samprapti Lakshanayoho Sambandah,* even though this concept was present since antiquity. The same pattern is employed to describe samprapti (pathogenesis) of Pakshaghata in this book. The following are the ghataka (components) participating in the samprapti (pathogenesis) of this disease.

1. **Udbhavastana (Abode of Origin) :** Pakwashaya (Colon) is the udbhavastana (abode of origin) for all the Vatavyadhis.

Pakwashaya samutta grahanena sarve vatajaha
(Cha.vi.6/2 Chakrapani)

The factors promoting Vata, originating from the Vatakaraka nidana (etiological factors of Vata), get vitiated in this abode of its origin (Pakwashaya) and then helps in vitiating and promoting stanika (provincial) Vata dosha in the rogadhistana (abode of the disease) – Mastishka (Brain) through rasayani (nutrient conduits). It is essential to know the udbhavastana (abode of origin) from the standpoint of treatment.

2. **Dosha (Vitiator):** Pakshaghata (Hemiplegia), has been since considered as one among Vata nanatmaja vyadhi (disease caused exclusively by Vata). (Ch.su.20/11), it is clear that the predominant dosha responsible for the disease is Vata. Its lakshanas (signs and symptoms) remain relevant to the lakshanas (signs and symptoms) of Vata. However, it is important for us to ponder as to which among five Vatas beginning with Prana, is responsible as a causative factor for Pakshaghata. Answer to this question has to be determined on the basis of the lakshanas (signs and symptoms) of this disease.

Kritsnordhakayaha tasya syat akarmanyo vichetanaha (Ma.ni.vyakhya)
Yada prakupito……tada anyatara pakshasya (su.su. 1\60-61)

Karmahani (loss of functions) pertaining to the hand and feet confined to one side is the dominant feature of this disease. Both hands and feets are karmendriyas (organs of execution).

Tadyata shrotr twak …hastopasta …pada
Tatra poorvani …..itarani panchakarmendriyani
(Su.sh.1/4)

Both these karmendriyas (organs of execution) would have lost the dharana shakti (sustaining power) to lift and hold horizontally to the ground against the gravitational force. The power to hold in this manner can be called dharana shakti (sustaining power). Since the dharana shakti (power to sustain) is weakened, hands and legs cannot be lifted and held fast. Such dharana shakti (power to sustain) of the karmendriyas (organs of execution) is derived from Pranavayu. When Pranavayu becomes aggravated the dharana shakti (power to sustain) of the indriyas (organs of execution) may become depleted or destroyed.

Pranotra murdhaga…\bhudhi hrdaya indriya chittadhrk
(A.h.su.12\4)

Dr. Sadashiva Sharma opines that though these activities are depleted it is not because of depletion in Vata but because of enhancement of Vata. Meaning one can understand that there is enhancement of Vata in the mastishka (brain) which is the adhishtana (abode) of vikrti (abnormality) and depletion of Vata at the vyaktistana (realm of manifestation).

Therefore, Pranavayu also is one of the components in the samprapti (pathogenesis) of Pakshaghata. Apart from these hands and feet would have lost the functions of utkshepana (adduction) apakshepana (abduction), grahana (grasping), dharana (sustaining) and gamana (movement) etc. Normal functioning of these activities, require Vyana vayu to remain normal. When it becomes aberrated, these activities also become impoverished or aberrant.

Vyano..../gatyapakshepanotkshepa.../Prayaha sarvaha kriyaha / (A.hr.su12/6-7)

Hence it can be said that Vyana vayu is also a component in the samprapti (pathogenesis) of this disorder.

Apart from this another type of Vata is also vikrta (abnormal) in this disorder. That is the Udana vata. In Pakshaghata for performance of the functions of Bahu (upper arm) and Uru (thigh) prayatna (effort) and bala (strength) are essential. The debilitations present in these two in this disorder can be known by akarmanyata (inertness in the activity) of the hand and the leg. Therefore, Udana vayu is a component in the samprapti (pathogenesis) of this disorder.

"Urastanamudanasya..vakpravrtihi prayatnorjabala... (A.h. su12/5) (prayatnaha)... karyeshu padarta grahanadishoodyamaha (A.da)

Association with Pitta causes Vatapittaja, association with Kapha causes Vatakaphaja Pakshaghata. In general, it can be said that association with Pitta or Kapha is present in most of the Pakshaghatas. Pitta can cause mastishka vidradi (cerebral abcess), through daha (inflammation) and paka (suppuration) because of its ushna (hot) and teekshna (fiery) properties. Puyotpati (purulence) is not possible in vidradhi (abscess) without Kapha. Therefore, Kapha is indispensable to the occurrence of mastishka vidradi (cerebral abscess). Not only that Kapha is essential for occurrence of mastishka arbuda (tumours of the brain). In this manner for the occurrence of mastishka vidradi (cerebral abscess) and raktasrava (hemorrhage), etc. Pitta and for the occurrence of tumours etc. Kapha are the causative factors. In this manner these two become indirectly responsible for mastishkagata margavarana (occlusion of cerebral conduit).

3. **Ama (Unaccomplished incompletely digested nutrient that is toxic)**: Ama, formed because of guru (heaviness) manda (inane) etc. properties of Kapha or because of the ksheenata (feebleness) of ushna (hot) and teekshna (fiery) properties of Pitta causing jataragnimandya (depleted combustive power of digestion) creates mastishkagata sira margavarana (occlusion of cerebral arteries) in turn resulting in aggravation of Vata. (Obstruction to the channels is one among the aftermath of occurrence of ama – *srotorodha balabhramsha gauravanila mudata*). Arbuda (tumours), Vidradi (abscess), Thrombosis etc. which can cause mastishkagata margavarana (obstruction to cerebral circulation) results from the respective *dhatvagnimandyajanya* (depleted combustive power of respective supportive elements causing) ama. On the whole in the samprapti (pathogenesis) of this disease, the role of ama formed by dhatvagnimandya (attenuation of combustive power) of rakta (blood), mamsa (flesh), meda (adipose tissue) and majja (marrow) is paramount.

4. **Sancharastana (Domain of Drift):** The vitiated Vata from the domain of accrual (sanchita stana) [i.e.: Pakwashaya (colon) which is also the udbhava stana (domain of origin)] travels to Mastishka (Brain) which is the rogadhistana (abode of disease) through rasayani (nutrient conduits)

5. **Adhistana (Abode)**: For every disease for its origin there is a specialized location.It is at this location that sroto dushti (vitiation of conduits) and dosha dushya sammurchana (coalescence of vitiator and defilable supportive element) occur. This kind of specialized location is called rogadhistana (abode of ailment). Pakshaghata (Hemiplegia) also must have such a specialized adhishtana (abode). Even though classics do not clearly pinpoint this location anywhere, in modern sciences it has been narrated that Hemiplegia (Hemiplegia has been correlated to Pakshaghata beforehand) has its abode in one part of the Mastishka (Brain) .

Harrison's Textbook of Medicine mentions that this disease occurs because of an aberration in any one half of the cerebral hemisphere (Hemiplegia is the classic sign of vascular disease and occurs chiefly with lesion of either cerebral hemisphere). This makes it clear that in this disease the abode of aberration lies in one part of the brain. What is the concept of Ayurveda in this context? We will ponder over this now.

One cannot sit with one's eyes closed as if it is not related to us just because this topic has not been mentioned in Ayurveda. Since it is possible to adopt a localized treatment and thereby benefit the patient by understanding the abode of disease, it is appropriate to comprehend it. With this discernment a modest effort has been made in the following passages to determine the rogadhistana (abode of disease) based on the concepts of Ayurveda.

Previously while discussing the role of doshas (vitiator) it has been mentioned that there is vitiation of Pranavayu. Moordha (vertex) is cardinal among the abodes of Pranavayu. (*stanam pranasya murdhoraha ...Ch.Chi 28/5)*. There is a reference at one point in Atharva veda that "(*Pavamano adhishirshitaha*)" (*A.kri.sha*) meaning vayu is localized in the adhisheersha (vertex of head). Many of the scholars have inferred the word adhisheersha mentioned here as cerebral cortex. While describing the abode of vayu in Kashyapa samhita, it has been mentioned that majja dhatu (marrow) is the abode of vayu. (*Adho nabhyasti majjani vatastanam prachakshate – (Ka. sam. su. 27/10)*. Indirectly this carries the meaning that wherever there is majja dhatu (marrow), vayu also will be present there. According to Ayurveda, majja dhatu (marrow) is located within the asti (bone). Mastishka (brain) which is located within the shirahakapalasti (skull) is also to be taken as majja dhatu (marrow).

This in Ayurveda is denoted as "Mastulunga"– *"Mastulungo avileena ghrtakara mastaka majja"- (Dalhana su.sha 10/42)*. This carries the meaning that majja dhatu (marrow) which is known by the term mastulunga that lies within the skull (shirahakapalasti) is the adhistana (abode) of vayu. The above references and descriptions are given to indicate that mastishka is one among the adhistana (abodes) of prakrta Vata (normal Vata). However, if there is a vikrti (aberration) in this abode, whether it leads to vitiation of Vata is something to be currently pondered. It has been mentioned earlier that Drdabalacharya in Chapter 9 of siddhistana of Charaka samhita has explained as to what are the consequences of shirobhighata (trauma to the head). Most of the aberrations described there pertain to Vata vikara (vitiation of Vata) and among them cheshtanasha and sanjnanasha (loss of activity and loss of consciousness) draw our attention in the present context. Both these lakshanas (symptoms) are seen in Pakshaghata and these two are also positively symptoms of Pranavikrti (aberrant Prana) – meaning when there is a Shiromarmabhighata (trauma to the vital center head) Pranavayu which has its adhistana (abode) there gets aggravated and its normal functions of indriya dharana (sustenance to sense organs) and chitta dharana (sustenance to mind) gets distorted. This results in akarmanyata (inactivity) and vichetanata (loss of consciousness). It is pertinent to clarify one more point here. Among the 107 marmas (vital points) there is no marma by name shiromarma. All marmas (vital poimts) located in the shirobhaga (region of head) are shiromarma only. There is no mention anywhere as to trauma to which of these marmas can cause Pakshaghata. It is not correct to argue that trauma to any one of these can cause Pakshaghata. At present we can only say that it is a subject matter for further research. Further, the word aghata (trauma) commonly assumes the meaning of bahyabhighata (external trauma). Here, since if there is an internal trauma to the doshas of shiro marma it can lead to Pakshaghata it is inevitable to extend the purview of the word aghata (trauma). Such an extended meaning of vyapti (pervasive) has been cognized here.

The notion that in Pakshaghata mastishka (brain) is the adhistana (abode) of vikrti (aberration) finds favourable support in the classical context during the narration of Pakshagata chikitsa (treatment of Pakshaghata) in Sushruta samhita. There describing the specialized treatment for Pakshagata it has been said "vaisheshikaschaatra *mastishkyaha shirobastihi" (Su.chi.5/19).*

Shirobasti (cumulative medicament to the head) and mastishkya (a procedure that provides nutrition to the brain) both are localized forms of treatment procedures carried out in the shiraha pradesha (region of the head). We can guess that Sushratacharya must have advocated the employment of these two localized treatments in particular, since he was aware that the adhistana (abode) of vikrti (aberration) probably lies in the Mastishka (Brain) .

Similarly, in many of the classical texts while describing as to how to employ Mahamasha taila in Pakshaghata, it has been indicated that procedures of karnapurana (instillation in the ear) and nasya (instillation in the nose) should be carried out with that oil. From this, it can be inferred that these two lines of treatments have been specifically prescribed since the adhistana of vikrti (abode of aberration) lies somewhere in the mastishka (brain) that is close to ear (karna) and nose (nasa). The gist of all the above references - make it logically apparent that the moolaadhistana (source abode) of vikrti (aberration) in Pakshaghata lies somewhere in one portion of the mastishka (brain).

The centre for controlling the functions of hands and legs lies separately, both in the right and left hemispheres of the mastishka (brain). The nerves departing from this centre gets interchanged (decussation) at sushumna sheersha (medulla oblongata) resulting in the ones originating from the right hemisphere proceeding towards the left side and those originating from the left hemisphere proceeding towards the right side until they reach the anterior horn cells of sushumna (spinal cord). From there, they proceed towards the respective parts of the body. Therefore, the cardinal symptoms of Pakshaghata are seen on the contralateral side to the side of vikrti (aberration) in the mastishka (brain). When there is vikrti (aberration) in the centre of the brain that controls both hand and feet movements there is loss of function in both hands and feet or since these two nerves pass very closely in the internal capsule, vikrti (aberration) in this area results in loss of function in the hand and feet. Most of the Pakshaghata results from vikrti (aberration) at this region. This is diagrammatically displayed. The nerves relating to the face originate from the front of the above-mentioned centers. Therefore, if the extent of vikrti (aberration) is not that extensive there will be no deformity in the face. Apart from this both left and right sides of the trunk of the body receive nerves from two sides of the brain. Therefore, the functions of the trunk of the body will continue through nerves of the normal half even if there is vikrti (aberration) in one side of the mastishka (brain). (The loss of functions seen in the hand and the feet will not be seen on that side of the trunk of the body).

6. **Dushya (Defilable Sustaining Elements):** This chapter on dushya is intended to deliberate on dhatu (supportive elements),upadhatu (subsidiary supportive elements) and mala (defilements) that take part in the causation of the disease.

While describing the samprapti (pathogenesis) of the disease, it is stated "*sira,snayurvishoshya cha*" (A.h.ni15/38-39) indicating that sira (arteries) and snayu (muscles) are emaciated.If not in all the contexts at least in the present context the word sira should be used to cognize the dhamani (arteries) and not veins alone. When siradushti is viewed with this meaning it can be said that the causative factors of Pakshaghata such as those described in the modern medicine - atherosclerosis, hypertension, thrombosis, embolism etc. are different varieties of siradushti (arterial vitiation). Most of these mentioned here before, cause occlusion in the conduits of mastishkagata sira (cerebral arteries) and consequent Vata prakopa (aggravation of Vata) or the hemorrhage that occurs by dissection of wall of the blood vessels in the brain as a result of hypertension can also be taken as a type of siradushti (arterial vitiation). From another standpoint siradushti (arterial vitiation) is meaningful in Pakshaghata. Even in modern medicine Hemiplegia has been considered as a cerebrovascular disease. This is supportive of the concept of siradushti (arterial vitiation) in Pakshaghata as narrated in Ayurveda. Apart from this it is clear that this knowledge was present thousands of years before modern medicine cognized this fact. Sira are the upadhatu (subsidiary supportive elements) of rakta "*Asrjaha khandaraha siraha*". Raktadushti (vitiation of blood) can cause siradushti (vitiation of arteries). Due to this the sira (walls of the cerebral arteries) become brittle, causing internal hemorrhage, thereby causing avarana (girdling) of the Vata present in that location resulting in the possibility of Pakshaghata. The emaciation of muscles narrated in the samprapti (pathogenesis) will have to be explained by observing the status of the mamsa peshi (muscles) of the affected hand and feet of the patient. Vatavaha nadi have been denoted as snayu in Vaidyaka shabda sindhu "*snayuhu stree klee vayuvaha nadyam*". In this context the word snayu if assumed to mean Vatavaha nadi then it will not be wrong to assume that the composite word snayu vishoshana (emaciation of snayu) can mean the vikrti (aberration) of

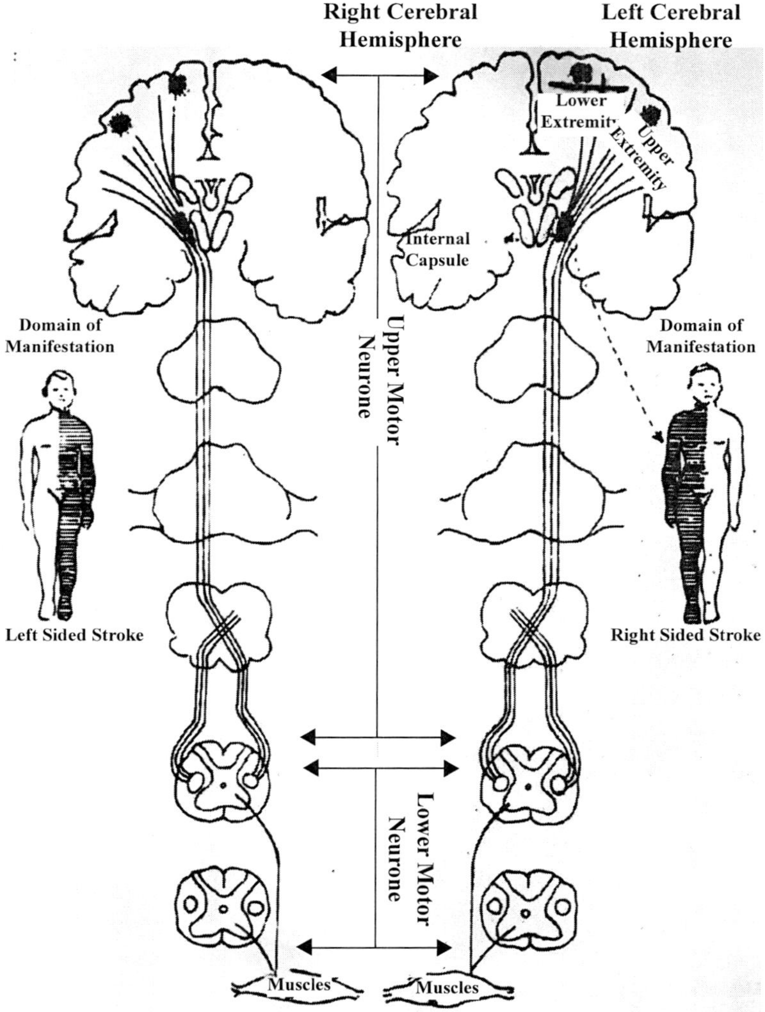

- Indicates Points of Lesion

Diagram Showing the Brain and the Lesions in Pakshaghata (Hemiplegia)

nadi (defective functioning of nerves innervating the muscles of the affected side) related to the muscles of the hand and feet resulting in the weakness or emaciation of muscles. Not only this the common meaning of snayu is a variety of mamsa peshi. This is of 4 types.

1. Prtanavati(Ramifying and branching)
2. Vrttha (Ring shaped)
3. Prtu (Thick or broad)
4. Sushira (perforated)

(Su.sha 5/30-34)

Extremities (hands and legs) contain Prtanavati snayu. The role of snayu (muscles) is to provide the ability to carry weight. “Snayubhihi bahubhirbaddhaha tena bhara sahaha naraha”. In Pakshaghata since the muscles of the hand and feet of the affected side of the patient gets emaciated, the hand and feet of the aberrant half of that patient do not have the strength to bear weight. This can be assumed as a symptom of snayu vishoshana (emaciation of muscles). It is essential to view the vishoshana (emaciation) of sira (arteries) and snayu (muscles) from the standpoint of their origin also. It has been said that these two originate from the sneha (oleaginous) part of medas (adiposity).

“ Medasaha snehamadaya sirasnayutwamapnuyat
Siranam tu mrduhupakaha snayunam cha tataha kharaha
“(Su.sha.7/28)

Ruksha (dry) and Khara (rough) food as well as living habits that aggravates Vata causes depletion in the snehamsha (unctuousness) of sira (arteries) and snayu (muscles) desiccating these two, consequent to the depletion of snehamsha (unctuousness) of medas (adipose tissue). The snayu (muscles) [deficiently nourished by unctuosity of medas (adipose tissue)] become vishushka (desiccated), are weak causing deficiency in functions of bhara vahana (bearing weight) dharana (sustaining) etc. From the description it is clear that the three pradhana dhatu (cardinal supportive elements) rakta,mamsa and medas; two cardinal upadhatus (subsidiary supportive elements) sira and snayu take part in the samprapti (pathogenesis) of Pakshaghata. Apart from this the majja dhatu (marrow) also coordinates in the samprapti (pathogenesis) of this roga in its own specialized manner. This subject has been narrated during the discussion of adhishtana (abode) heretofore.

7. **Srotas (Systems) :** This is a disease pertaining to the Vatavaha srotas (System). Since in this disease there is the context of vitiation of raktavaha sira srotas [vascular system] this disease can be assumed to occur because of raktavaha srotodusti (vitiation of cerebro vascular system) in the mastishka (brain) which is one of the stana (abodes) of Vata. The variety of srotodusti here is mainly of sangha (obstruction).

8. **Vyakti Stana (Domain of Manisfestation)**- Vama/ Dakshina parshva (Left or right half) .

The components of samprapti (pathogenesis) described so far can be summarized as follows.

i. **Udbhava Stana (Abode of Origin)**: Pakwashaya

ii. **Dosha (Vitiator)**: Mainly Prana vayu

Udana and Vyana also have a role. Sometimes Kapha or Pitta can be associated.

iii. **Ama (Unaccomplished incompletely digested nurient that is toxic)** - Ama originating from jataraghni and dhatvagni

iv. **Sanchara stana (Domain of Drift)**- Rasayani (Nutrient conduits)

v. **Adhishtana (Abode)** - one specific part of the mastulunga or mastishka (brain)

vi. **Dushya (Domain of Defilement)** - Rakta (blood), Mamsa (flesh), Medas (adipose) and Majja (marrow) Dhatu (supportive elements)); Sira (arteries) and Snayu (muscles)

vii. **Srotas (Systems)** - Mainly Vatavaha and Raktavaha

viii. **Srotodushti Prakara (Type of Vitiation of Systems)** - Predominantly sanga (obstructive)

ix. **Vyakti stana (Domain of Manifestation)** - Left or right upper/lower extremities.

Vatakara nidana (etiological factors aggravating Vata)
(food and living habits)

↓

Accumulation of Vata in Pakwashaya (large intestine) -
(**Sanchayavasta**)

↓

Continued devouring of nidana (etiological factors)

↓

Vata gets ready to move to different parts of the body from Pakwashaya - (**Prakopavasta** – Stage of Aggravation)

↓

Repeated indulgence in the nidana (etiological factors) and non-expulsion of accumulated Vata

↓

Vata that has become Unmarga gamitva (upwardly mobile) moves towards the brain through the rasayani (nutrient conduits) - (**Prasaraavasta** - Stage of drift)

↓

Sangha (Occlusion) of vitiated Vata at a part of the brain where there is Khavaigunya (aberration of conduits) - (**Stana samshrayavasta** - Stage of accrual)

↓

Provincial dosha - Pranavayu vikrti, Vyanavayu vikrti resulting in sira (arteries) snayu (muscles) shosha (emaciation).

↓

Loss of function in the organs of execution (karmendriya) such as hands and feet - **Vyaktavasta** (Stage of manifestation)

Sankhya Samprapti of Pakshaghata

(Numerical Classification of Pathogenesis of Pakshaghata)

So far, Vikalpa samprapti has been described among the different types of samprapti such as Sankhya, Vikalpa etc. Among the remaining types of samprapti, Sankhya samprapti has been explained in the tabular form below. From this it can be understood as to how many types of samprapti (pathogenesis) are possible in Pakshaghata by a meticulous study of nidana, etc. (etiology, etc.)

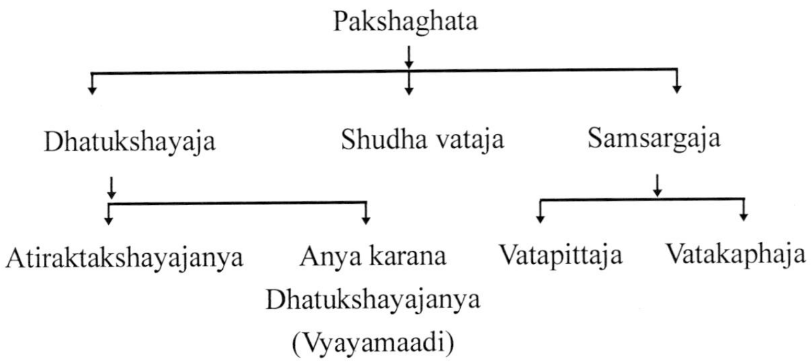
Pakshaghata
Dhatukshayaja
Shudha vataja
Samsargaja
Atiraktakshayajanya
Anya karana Dhatukshayajanya (Vyayamaadi)
Vatapittaja
Vatakaphaja

CHAPTER – 6

Purvarupa – Rupa Prakarana

Treatise on Prodromal Signs - Symptoms and Signs and Symptoms

Specific Purvarupa (Prodromal signs and symptoms) for Pakshaghata have not been mentioned in the classical texts. While describing the samanya Purvarupa (general Prodromal signs-symptoms) of Vata roga, it has been mentioned that if the signs and symptoms of specific Vata rogas are present in incipient and unmanifested form such should be considered as the Purvarupa (Prodromal signs-symptoms) of relevant Vata roga. Here avyakta rupa (unmanifested signs and symptoms) should be understood as those incipient or vaguely manifested symptoms. In other words where the signs and symptoms of Pakshaghata are incipient or vague, it should be understood as Purvarupa (Prodromal signs-symptoms). Apart from this, in some patients, shirashula (headache), bhrama (giddiness) and tama pravesha (transient syncope) can also be understood as Purvarupa (Prodromal signs-symptoms). Other than this those that are commonly seen as purvavasta (antecedent phases) of staana samshraya (accrual at a locus) such as aatopa (borborygmus) in purely Vataja Pakshaghata, osha (burning), chosha (heat) and paridaha (consummate burning) in Pitta samsargaja (conjoined with pitta) Pakshaghata and aruchi (tastelessness), avipaka (indigestion), angasada (heaviness of limbs) and chardi (vomiting) in Kapha samsargaja (conjoined with kapha) Pakshaghata can also be viewed as Purvarupa (Prodromal signs and symptoms) of Pakshaghata.

Rupa (Signs and Symptoms) or Lakshanas (Attributes)

These are seen during the fifth stage of samprapti (pathogenesis). Based on available classical literature in Ayurveda the following descriptions should be understood as lakshanas (attributes) of Pakshaghata.

A) Pratyatma lakshana (Cardinal Attribute) –

1. **Hasta karmahani (Impairment of Functions of Hand)** – Hand is one among the karmendriyas (organs of execution). Aberrations occurring in the mastishka (brain) which is the abode of karmendriya (organs of execution) results in impairment in functions of the hand correlating to the vikrta parshwa (aberrant flank). Mula granta's (core texts) mention the occurrence of akarmanyata (inertness) of the hand. Akarmanyata (inertness) has been clarified by the commentator of Madhu kosha (akarmanya ishath cheshta kshamaha) and Dalhana (akarmanya ishath karma kshayam) as alpa karyakshama (meagre functional ability) – meaning that there need not be complete loss of function of the hand. Deficiency in the functions of the hand can also be construed as impairment of hand function (hasta karma hani). Normal function of the hand comprises grahana (grasping) and dharana (sustaining). The physician should hold a pen or

pencil in his hand by the fingers and instruct the patient to pull it towards himself holding by the fingers of the vikrta parshwa (impaired flank). If the grahana shakti (grasping power) of the fingers of the hand is normal he will be able to pull towards himself with a power equal to the power of the physician's hand. If not, he will not be able to hold. Attempts to pull towards himself will be feeble. His grahana shakti (grasping power) can also be examined by asking the patient to unbutton his shirt or if he knows how to write, by asking him to write with a pen, etc.

The Patient should be told to lift the hand of the aberrant flank and hold it horizontal to the ground. When the dharana shakti (sustaining power) is depleted, he will not be able to lift and hold it horizontal to the ground. The depletion in grahana (grasping) and dharana (sustaining) shakti (power) of hand can be understood by aforementioned methods. In this context it has been mentioned in Charaka samhita that there will be cheshta nivrti (loss of mobility) of hands and feet. Cheshta nivrti means a variety of multifold functions of the hand gets debilitated or lost. The cheshta nivrti (loss of mobility) of the arms can be understood by asking the patient to touch his thumb by different fingers (fingers of the same hand) or touch different fingers of the same hand with the thumb, by asking the patient to flex and extend all the fingers and by asking the patient to do utkshepana (abduction), apakshepana (adduction), akunchana (flexion), prasarana (extension), gamana (movement) and vyavartana (rotation), etc. functions of the arm. Vitiation of Vyana vayu and Udana vayu are the cause for cheshta nivrti (loss of mobility). According to the modern physician emeritus Mr. Saville, in Hemiplegia aberration of hand is more pronounced than aberration of feet. More so, the mobility of the distal parts of the extremities (fingers of the hand). (The arm is affected more than the leg and the distal movements suffer more than the proximal ones- Saville).

Even though it is not narrated precisely in Ayurveda that loss of grasping power is more pronounced at the distal part, it stands to common logic that the opinion expressed in Ayurveda that there will be grahana karmahani (loss of grasping power) leads to the construal that distal part of the arm has become aberrant.

Expediting on the topic, Saville opines that if the patient is unconscious, by lifting each of the extremities of the patient and dropping it, the loss of function of the extremity should be determined by the intensity of the speed with which the extremity batters against the ground. (If the patient is conscious, we recognize the paralysis by lifting the limbs and letting them drop in turn-Saville). The dharana karmahani (loss of sustaining function) of the arms can be understood through the above procedure. The other characteristics described by him have been highlighted underneath in original form since they comprise an admirable description of cheshta nivrti (loss of mobility) explained in our classics.

"In slighter cases, weakness of dorsiflexion of the wrist and clumsiness of fine finger movements can be observed.

The upper limb is held with arm adducted at the shoulder and flexed at the elbows, wrist and fingers, with the forearm slightly pronated" (Saville).

The above description can be seen in the diagrams below.

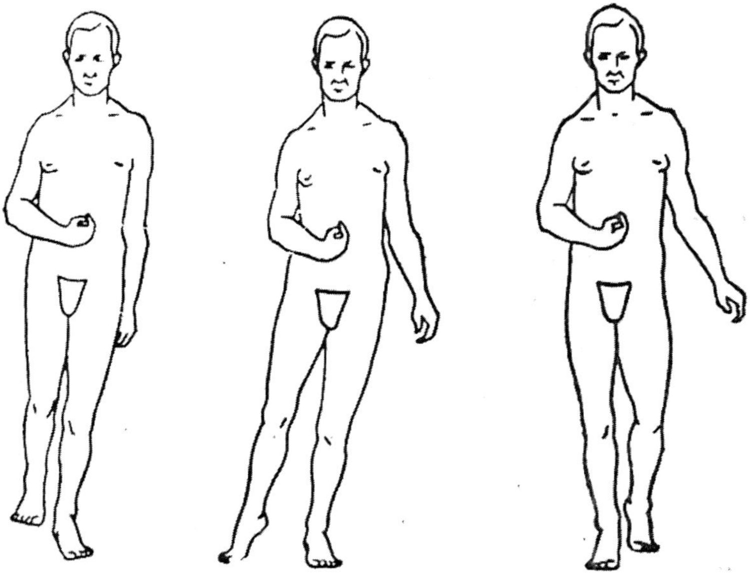

2. **Pada karmahani (Impairment of Functions of Feet)** –Gamana (locomotion) or walking is the main function of feet as a sense organ.

"Padau gamana karmani "(Ch. sha. 5/ 25-26)

Each individual based on his prakrti (constitution) has varied types of gamana swarupa (locomotory modality)

(e.g.: ...saragatayo na skalanti, adhishtitagatarveyaha sana padena mahim akramanti...Cha.sam.vi.8/66 Chakrapani).

This is normal. This normal gait alters in a patient of Pakshaghata and he walks in a distinctive '*hemiplegic gait*'. Patient strides hauling his crippled leg through a semi-circle. In this process, the toe of the feet will be extended towards the floor. He walks without bending the leg (in the extended form) at the vamkshana sandhi (hip joint) and janu sandhi (knee joint). The muscles of the leg facilitating flexion at janu (knee) and vamkshana (hip) sandhi (joint) become weak. Hence patient finds it difficult to flex the janu vamkshana sandhi (knee and hip joints). But flexing of the feet, at gulfa sandhi (ankle joint), can happen easily. The gait of this patient is described in the text "clinical examination in neurology", in these lines - "Most upper motor neuron lesions will produce an increase in muscular tone and will give rise to a spastic gait. When this is unilateral as in the case of hemiparetic, the affected limb is moved forward with difficulty occasioned by the lack of freedom of movement in all the joints. In addition, the toe of the affected extremity tends to be forced downward. This necessitates an abduction and circumduction of the limb in order to move it forward quickly. So, the toe of the shoe is dragged and may be noticeably worn on the outer aspect". The explanations given above can depict pada karma kshaya (infirmity of the feet) or cheshta nivrti (loss of mobility) as described in our classics. The gait can be seen in the given diagram above.

B) Samanya Lakshanas (Common Attributes)–

1. **Vichetanata (Loss of Consciousness)** – In certain contexts vichetanata carries the meaning of sparsha vikrti (aberrant touch). Sparsha vikrti (aberrant touch) is very rare

in this disease. Therefore, it is more appropriate to understand vichetanata here as unconsciousness. Chetanavasta (state of consciousness) implies a status of the soul (atma) accompanied by the indriyas (sense organs) capable of arta grahana (material cognition).

Sendriyam chetanam proktam (Cha.su.1)

Even though accompanied by such sense organs, in states of sushupti (deep sleep) and swapnavasta (sleep with dreams), the atma (soul) typically does not gain knowledge of indriyarta (sense objects). This is a normal jaivika pratikriya (sentient response). The state of deprivation of knowledge to the soul due to any reason through any of the sense organs (five sense organs), apart from the aforementioned circumstances, can be called the state of vichetanavasta (insentience) or murcha (unconsciousness). This kind of vichetanata (insentience) can be seen as a symptom during the early stages of Arterial obstruction, Thrombosis, and Hemiplegia due to Mastishkagata raktasrava (intracerebral hemorrhage). It is difficult to believe that ancient acharyas had failed to perceive a symptom that is predominantly seen during the early stages. Having noticed this, they might have used the term vichetana (insentience) for murcha (unconsciousness). Commentators have narrated "*vichetano alpachetanaha eeshath sparshadi jnanavanityartaha*" (Madhukosha). Alpa chetana (meagre sentience) means existence of sparsha vijnana (knowledge of tactility) etc. to a lesser extent meaning unconsciousness is not so grave. This is essentially true in this disease. Starting with onset of agambhira murchavasta (trivial unconsciousness) later on impaired movements and other symptoms come into manifestation. Unconsciousness will be very transient. It has been pointed out by Dalhana in this regard that if the patient is unconscious death may also occur.

"achetanam alpachetanam...yada achetanam bhavati tada asoon pranan parityajati"

2. **Ruja (Ache) or Vedana (Pain)** – In most of the patients of Pakshaghata ache or pain is not manifested on the aberrant side. There is no reference to pain in Hemiplegia in modern medical science. However, pain has been observed (by experience) in the aberrant extremities particularly at the root of the arm, in a minority of the patients. In some others this disease commences with the onset of a headache. It has to be conjectured that those classical authors have proclaimed this very symptom as 'pain'.

3. **Vak stambha (Stalling of Speech): -** Vak stambha means stalling of speech. In the process of modulation of speech jihva (tongue), kanta (throat), mukha kuhara (buccal cavity) and Udana vayu have a cardinal role. Tongue is a karmendriya (sensory organ of execution). [It is also the abode of rasanendriya (olfactory sense organ)]. Vak stambha (stalling of speech) occurs because of vitiation of adhistana of karmendriya (the abode of sensory organ of execution) as well as vitiation of Udana vayu. Udana vayu is a form of Vata responsible for vak pravrti (performance of speech). Vak sthambha (stalling of speech) is the result of its vitiation. Normal movement of the tongue as an organ does not occur. To know whether there is aberration of tongue or not, patient should be made to extend the tongue outward, move it to left

and right direction, to touch different parts [danta (teeth), oshta (lips), talu (palate) etc)] inside the mouth, as well as to utter some sounds. Vak stambha (stalling of speech) need not always be Vak stabdha (Aphasia – complete cessation of speech). Even if there is aspashta (dysphasia - incoherent) and krchra (dysarthria – difficult) shabdocharana (articulation of speech) it is appropriate to know this as Vak stambha in the present context. This type of speech impediment vak krchrate (dysarthria – difficult articulation of speech) can be cognized as the patient narrates his history itself. This is more commonly seen in right sided stroke. This is because speech centres are located in the left hemisphere of the brain. (Speech centers are not there in the right hemisphere of brain). This symptom is seen if there is aberration in the speech center along with that of center for control of hands and legs in the left hemisphere.

C) Anushangika Lakshana (Concomitant Attributes)–

1. **Snayu-peshi Shosha (Emaciation of Muscles-tendons): -** The Pratanavati muscular tendons located in the aberrant extremities get emaciated in course of time more than the normal muscles of extremities. Shosha (emaciation) is one among the aberrant acts of Vata such as sramsa (disintegration)– vyasadi (cleaving, etc). Since there is vitiation of Vata, shosha (emaciation) which is its aberrant act manifests in the muscles in course of time. This can be understood through inspection.

2. **Mamsa peshi stabdata (Inertness of Muscles)**– This is the combined effect of ruksha (dryness) and parushya (sternness). Flexion ensues at manibandha (wrist) and

kurpara sandhi (elbow joints). If the physician tries to extend such flexed joints (passive extension), extension will not occur easily.

There will be resistance by the muscles.

D) Samsargika lakshanas (Associated Attributes): Based upon samprapti (pathogenesis) and lakshanas (attributes), Pakshaghata can be said to be mainly of two types.

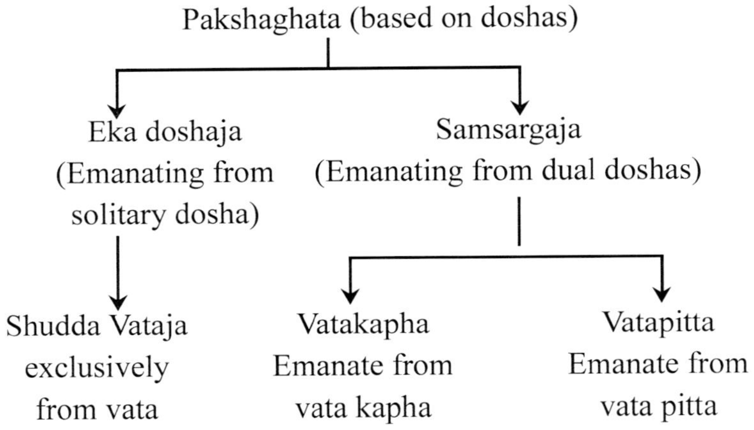

Affiliated with the signs and symptoms described so far, some unique signs and symptoms based on samsargika (associated) doshas come into manifestation. They are described here –

Signs and Symptoms Emanating from Vata Pitta –

1) **Daha (Burning)** – Aatura jneya (experienced by the patient) in the aberrant extremities.

2) **Santapa (Warmth)** – Sparsha jneya (experienced by palpation) – in the aberrant extremities.

3) **Murcha (Unconsciousness)**

Signs and Symptoms Emanating from Vata Kapha

1) **Shaitya (Coldness)** – Sparsha jneya (experienced by palpation)– in the aberrant extremities.

2) **Shota (Swelling)** – Darshana jneya (recognized by inspection) – in the aberrant extremities.

3) **Guruta (Heaviness)** – Experienced by the patient – in the aberrant extremities.

It should be understood that Pakshaghata is caused exclusively emanating from Vata if signs and symptoms enumerated from A) to C) are alone present without aforementioned samsargaja (composite) signs and symptoms.

Daha santapa murchasyuhu vayau pitta samanvite shaitya shota gurutwani tasminnevate kaphanvite shudha vata hatam paksham (Ma.ni. 22/42-43).

Pakshaghata due to rakta kshaya (diminution of blood) and Pakshaghata resulting from dhatu kshaya (diminution of sustaining factors) due to a variety of causes manifest attributes of Shudha Vataja (emanating exclusively from Vata) Pakshaghata itself.

The changes that occur in the signs and symptoms of the patient after the commencement of the treatment ensue in a specific sequence. Physicians should be aware of the specific sequence of changes that occur in the signs and symptoms to appreciate whether the treatment being given is efficacious or not. From this standpoint signs and symptoms can be classified into two phases –

I. Stage of Onset –

a. Udara pratyavartana kriya (abdominal reflexes) are lost.

b. The pada pratyavartana kriya usually have urdhvamukhaprasarana of toes (plantar reflexes commonly have extension of toes from the beginning).

c. Trunk muscles are weakened on the affected side.

d. During the early few hours, the janu pratyavartana kriya (reflex action of the knee) is lost and subsequently within the first 10 days become hyperactive.

II. Parivartanavasta (Stage of Transformation) –

a. Initially the flexor group of muscles of the arm develops strength.

b. Patient may become competent to lift his arm (adduction) and to move it away from his body (abduction) (movement mediated by axillary joint). Flexion becomes possible at kurpara (ankle), manibandha (wrist) and anguli (fingers).

c. In the legs prasaraka peshi samuha (extensor group of muscles) gain strength initially. Because of this the act of extension mediated by janu (knee) and vamkshana sandhi (hip joints) may return to complete normalcy. The power to bring the legs towards the body (power of adduction) return to complete normalcy. But it will not be possible to bend the feet upwards towards the thigh (dorsiflexion).

Besides the finer movements of the fingers of the feet will not be normal.

d. Urdva udara pratyavartana kriya (upper abdominal reflexes) return to normalcy earlier than Adho udara pratyavartana kriya (lower abdominal reflexes)

e. The response of Padatala pratyavartana kriya (plantar reflexes) will be of the nature of flexion. (From Saville's text)

CHAPTER – 7

Vyavachedaka Nidana – Sadhyasadhyata Prakarana Treatise on Differential Diagnosis – Prognostication

---

A gross attempt has been made in this chapter to understand in what other diseases and aberrant states the prime signs and symptoms such as loss of movement of the extremities is seen as in the case of Pakshaghata (Hemiplegia) and in what manner they are at variance from Pakshaghata. Diseases Pangu (lame), Khanja (monoplegia), Sarvanga roga (quadriplegia), Ekanga vata (monoplegia), Ardita vata (Bell's palsy) and Viswachi (Brachial neuralgia / palsy) to some extent resemble Pakshaghata. The differences seen between them have been listed side by side here below under respective disease headings.

Pakshaghata	**Pangu**
Functional impairment occurs in one leg and one hand of one flank.	Both legs are functionally impaired. Arms do not have impairment.
Originates from trauma to shiro marma (vital part of the head). Origin not due to trauma to kukundhara marma (vital point in the low back).	Probably originates from trauma to kukundhara marma (vital point in the low back).

Pakshaghata	**Pangu**
Probably not a janmabala pravrta vyadhi (congenital disease) Predominates during middle and and old age.	Possible that this is congenital. Predominates in childhood and adult.
From the standpoint of treatment easier to treat than janmabala pravrta Pangu (congenital paraplegia). [Excluding Pakshaghata due to kshaya).]	Impossible or more difficult than Pakshaghata.
Hemiplegia	Paraplegia.

Pakshaghata	**Khanja**
Functional impairment of one hand and one leg is inevitable.	Functional impairment of one leg only.
Probably there is no saktni khandara kshobha (inflammation of tendons of thigh)	Commonly thigh of the aberrant leg that is from gulfa (ankle) to janga (proximal part of thigh) become weak.
Not a janmabala pravrta vyadhi (congenital disease)	Mostly seen as janmabala pravrta vyadhi (congenital disease)
Hemiplegia	A type of Monoplegia

Pakshaghata	**Sarvanga Roga**
Functional impairment of the legs and hands of either left or right side.	Both extremities of both sides are functionally impaired.
There are chances of recovery even though with some difficulty.	Difficult to treat.
Hemiplegia	Quadriplegia

Pakshaghata	Ekangavata
Inevitably it is essential that one leg and one hand becomes functionally impaired.	One leg or One hand alone becomes aberrant. Both extremities of one side will not be aberrant.
Hemiplegia	Monoplegia.

Pakshaghata	Arditavata
Mukhardha vikrti confined only to lower half of the face, if at all present.	Mukhardha vikrti (aberration of one half of the face) is very essential.
Half of the body (one flank) only aberrant.	Aberration of one half of the face alone present. Functional impairment of the legs and hands of either left or right side is absent.
Hemiplegia	Bell's palsy (Facial paralysis)

Pakshaghata	Vishwachi
Not only functional impairment of hand (arm) but also functional impairment of the leg exists.	Exclusively functional impairment of arm. Functional impairment of leg will not be there.
Aberrant arm will be in an unusual attitude.	None
Functional impairment will be present only in one arm.	Functional impairment may be present in both arms.
Hemiplegia	Brachial neuralgia / palsy

Sometimes Viswachi can be present in the upper extremity of one side and there is possibility for the existence of Khanja in the lower extremity of the same side. In such instances suspicion may arise as to whether this is Pakshaghata (Hemiplegia) seeing the aberration manifested in the leg and hand unilaterally. Hence their differential diagnosis is given here.

Pakshaghata	**Vishwachi (left arm or right arm)** **Khanja (left leg or right leg)**
Functional impairment of one hand and leg of one side concurrently	Generally functional impairment of hand and feet is not concurrent.
Spastic gait is the predominant symptom of the disease.	Vikala gati (aberrant gait) [(anirdhista rupa) [non-specific form] is present.
As explained in hasta karmahani (functional impairment of the hand), the flexion of the kurpara (elbow), manibandha (wrist) and anguli sandhi (finger joints) are of unique kind.	Functional impairment of hand is predominant.

Vidyotini commentary in Hindi on Madhava nidana by Sri Sudarshana shastri has been taken as reference for the afore-mentioned nomenclatures of modern medicine.

In the preceding context of etiology (hetu) it was stated that Pakshaghata (Hemiplegia) occurs due to reasons of bleeding, etc. in the brain. Based on the attributes, to some extent, the internal causative factors can be understood. Hence vyavachedaka nidana (differential diagnosis) based on causes can be delineated as below.

Vyavachedaka Nidana (Differential Diagnosis) Based on Karana (Etiology)

Notable Features	Dhamani margavarodha(Arterial occlusions)	Thrombosis	Mastishkagata raktasrava (Cerebral Haemorrhage)
1. Age	Youth	Predominant during middle and old age	Preponderant during old age
2. Onset	Sudden	Gradual	Sudden with headache and vomiting
3. Previous historyof illness	Hrthkapatavikrti (Cardiac valvular diseases) Dhamani shota (Thrombo phlebitis) Asti bhagnajanya majja bahirgamana (Seepage of bonemarrow from fractures) (admixture with blood)	Dhamani katinya (Atherosclerosis) Upadamsha (Syphilis) etc.	Jeerna vrkkashota (Chronic nephritis) Madhumeha (Diabetes) Dhamani katinya (Atherosclerosis) etc

4. Shira shula (Headache)	Rare	Not present	Severe
5. Aakshepa (Convulsions)	Rare	Present	Not present
6. Murcha (Unconsciousness) and Sanyasa (Coma)	Agambira murcha (Shallow unconsciousness)	Gambira moorcha (Profound unconsciousness)	Gambira murcha (Profound unconsciousness) Sanyasa (Coma) Marana (Death)
7. Sheershambu (CSF)	Blood stained with excessive pressure	Clear Low pressure	Clear Normal pressure
8. Prognosis	Survives	Chances of survival present	Death is more common

Sadhyasadhyata (Prognosis)

Vatavyadhi is one among eight Maha roga (prodigious diseases)

(Vatavyadhihi pramehascha ...astakam (Su.sam.su.22/45).

Since the strength of the illness is more in these diseases, these diseases will not be subdued by ordinary or informal treatments. In these distinctive lines of treatment have to be followed for prolonged duration. That is why these are called Maha vyadhi (Prodigious illnesses). Pakshaghata (Hemiplegia) is one among the Vatavyadhi that is included under Maha vyadhi (Prodigious illnesses). In other words, Pakshaghata is a disease affiliated to Maha vyadhi (Prodigious illnesses). Therefore, this disease, from the standpoint of treatment naturally has a difficult prognosis.

It has been mentioned in Yogaratnakara that Vatavyadhis are difficult to treat and if cured it is only due to the good fortune of the patient and treatment should never be started in Vatavyadhi with a challenge that I will cure it definitely. Meaning Pakshaghata which is a Vata roga is difficult to treat. Yet if treatment is started reasoning that treating is one's singular duty without making a challenge, it can be said that it may be cured, due to the good fortune of the patient.

(vata rogastu asadhyo ayam daivayogat susidhyati / anumanena kurvanti vaidyakam na pratijnaya. (Yo.ra.vata roga)

From the standpoint of treatment till the time of classics of Yogaratnakara, (Seventeenth Century) Vata rogas were a challenging invitation to the physician. It is not an exaggeration to state that this status more or less remains the same even today. Hence Pakshaghata should not be viewed lightly from the standpoint of treatment.

According to Acharya Sushruta Pakshaghata emanating from Vata kapha and Vata pitta are sadhya (viable); Pakshaghata emanating exclusively from Vata is krichra sadhya (formidable) and it has been stated that Pakshaghata that is dhatu kshaya janya (genesis from diminution of dhatus) and raktatisrava janya (genesis from excessive hemorrhage) are asadhya (unviable).

(shudha vata hatam paksham krichrasadhyatamam viduhu/ sadhyamanyena samyuktam asadhyam kshaya hetukam // (Su.sam.ni.1/61)

Here Dalhanacharya narrates that according to Gayadasa 'kshaya hetuka' means *"shonitati sruta krta dhatukshayameva asadhyam //*

Same inference has been narrated above. In his commentary "Nyaya chandrika" Gayadasa has narrated that one should understand Pakshaghata arising from any cause other than dhatu kshaya (diminution of dhatus) due to raktasrava (hemorrhage) as krchra sadhya (formidable). (Su. sam.su.1/62)

In the above references two aspects have been mainly considered:

1) Dosha samsarga (Association of doshas)

2) Dhatu kshaya (Diminution of dhatu)

Acharya Charaka has mentioned that if Vatavyadi's are not correctly diagnosed in time or even if diagnosed relevant treatment is not provided in time and disregarded, or if the disease has become chronic by more than one year it is unviable or difficult to treat.

(*sarveshvete aparijnataha parisamvatsarastata /*
Upekshanadasadhyaha syuhu
Or
Durupakramaha – Cha.chi.28/235-236)

According to this reference the points to be observed are:

1) Proper diagnosis of the disease

2) Treatment at the right time

3) Duration of illness.

In another context in Charaka Samhita, Drdabalacharya has stated that Vatavyadi because of the gravity of their location (being localized in the brain) are very difficult to cure or are incurable: - apart from that if they are free from upadrava (supervenient afflictions), if the patient is robust and the disease is not chronic it can be cured through treatment.

(Yete stanasya gambhiryat yatnat sidhyanti va nava/
navan balavatastvetan sadhayet nirupadhravan/
Cha.sam.chi *28/-74)*

The prognosis stated for Vatavyadhi (aforementioned) is applicable for Pakshaghata as well.

According to this reference the points to be considered for determination of prognosis are:

1) Staana gambhirya (Locational gravity) - shiromarmadhistitadi (located in the vital centres of the head etc.)

2) Presence or absence of upadrava (supervenient afflictions).

3) Strength of the patient.

4) Duration of illness.

It has been stated above that presence or absence of upadrava (supervenient afflictions) helps in the determination of prognosis in Vata roga. Hence as to what are the upadrava (supervenient afflictions) of Vata roga can now be discerned. While narrating the upadrava (supervenient afflictions) of Vata roga, it has been said that, excluding the attributes of Vata roga, if any other attributes manifest such attributes are to be understood as upadrava (supervenient afflictions) of the respective Vata roga, or according to the opinion of Chakrapani Upadrava (supervenient afflictions) of avrta (girdled) Vata should be assumed as upadrava (supervenient afflictions) of Vata roga.

(Upadravaschatra shringagraahikaya anuktapi samanyopadrava lakshanayukta eva kechit gadaa vijneyaha; kimva adhyaya sheshe 'hridrogo vidradihi' ityadina vakshyamana upadrava jneyaha–

(Cha.sam.chi.28/74. Chakrapani)

Upadrava (supervenient afflictions) of avrta (girdled) Vata indicated by Chakrapani have been narrated in the following manner in Chapter 28 verse 236- 237 of Charaka chikitsa stana.

Hrdrogo vidradhihi pleeha gulmatisara evacha /
bhavanti upadravastesham avrtanam upekshanat /

Hrdroga (heart diseases), Vidradi (abscess), Pleeha roga (splenic disorders), Gulma (phantom tumors) and Atisara (diarrhea), manifest in the form of upadrava (supervenient afflictions) due to disregard of avrta (girdled) Vata. Chakrapani opines that this itself should be understood as upadrava (supervenient afflictions) of Vatavyadhi. Since Pakshaghata is a Vatavyadhi, aforementioned afflictions may come into manifestation here also.

Pakshaghata will not be cured if these upadrava (supervenient afflictions) manifest. If Hrdroga (heart diseases) in the form of upadrava (supervenient afflictions) occur it indicates the spread of doshas from one marma stana (vital site), [shiro marma (vital center of the head)] to another marma stana; upadrava (supervenient afflictions) such as Gulma (phantom tumor) and Atisara (diarrhea) indicate the spread of Pakshaghata dushti prabhava (defiling spell) from one roga marga (pathway of disease) [in Pakshaghata shiras (head) sira (arteries) snayu (muscles) are madhyama roga marga (intermediate disease pathways)] to another roga marga (path way of disease) [Gulma (phantom tumors) Atisara (diarrhea) are afflictions of abhyantara roga marga (internal path ways of disease)]. Vitiation of marma stana (vital sites) (due to diseases of heart, etc.) and manifestation of vitiation at more than one roga marga (disease pathway) – madhyama and abhyantara (intermediate and internal) are common attributes of incurability (Cha.sam.su. 10/11-20). Hence Pakshaghata may become incurable.

Based on an extraneous textual reference it has been stated in Madhava nidana that Pakshaghata is incurable if sparsha jnana (tactile sensation) becomes extinct in pregnant women, post-natal women, children, old age, debilitated and among those suffering from excessive blood loss due to whatever reason.

Garbhini sutika baalavrdhaksheeneshvasrksrute /
pakshaghatam pariharet vedanarahito yadi //
(Ma.ni.*Vatavyadhi)*

Apart from this, Pakshaghata is said to be incurable if accompanied with Visarpa (Erysipelas), Daha (burning sensation), Vedana (pain), Murcha (unconsciousness), Aruchi (lack of taste), Agnimandya (depleted digestive potential), Balaksheenata (physical weakness) and Mamsaksheenata (emaciated flesh). It is not clear here whether it is incurable if one or more of these upadrava (supervenient afflictions) are present or only if all the upadrava (supervenient afflictions) are present. Probably it becomes incurable if most among these upadrava (supervenient afflictions) are present. From the viewpoint of prognosis, the points observed in the above references are narrated herein.

1. Age: – baala (child) vrdha (senescent)
2. Certain natural states : – Garbhini (pregnant), Sootika (post-natal).
3. Upadrava (supervenient afflictions): – Visarpa (erysipelas), Murchadi (unconsciousness, etc.)
4. Bala (strength): – Ksheena bala (debilitated strength)

5. Dhatu stiti (status of dhatu): – Ksheena mamsa (emaciated flesh), Raktasravadi (hemorrhage etc)

6. Indriya stiti (sensory status): – Sparsha jnana heenata (depleted tactile sensation).

Ugradhityacharya, author of the text Kalyanakaraka has stated in a slightly different manner with regard to all other authors apropos prognosis of this disease. It is stated that sarvanga shota (generalized anasarca), sparsha rahitata (absent tactility), aadmana (tympanitis), bhagna (fractures), kampa (tremors), vedana rahitya (absence of pain sensation), mamsa shosha (emaciation of flesh) indicates incurability of Pakshaghata (Ka.kaa. 12/37)

Based on some Unani references the author of Chikitsa chandrodaya states that if the colour of skin remains unchanged, slightly thin and slightly edematous on the vikrta parshwa (aberrant side) the prognosis is good; excessive emaciation and discolouration of skin on the vikrta parshwa (aberrant side) is an indication of incurability (Chi.cham. sam.1). This is a somewhat odd opinion. This cannot be seen in any of the texts of Ayurveda or Modern medicine. This kind of discoloration of skin or oedema of the skin is not commonly observed in Pakshaghata. However, if this is helpful for prognostication it is desirable to cognize it.The prognosis according to Modern medicine is based on the svarupa (features) of samprapti (pathogenesis) of this disease. Harrison's Textbook of Medicine states-

"Prognosis of the stroke is probably due to increasing stenosis of the involved artery by neural thrombus or to extension of the thrombus along the artery to block side branches and hinder anastomic flow. In the case of large infarcts, swelling of the large infarcted tissue may occur, tentorial herniation follows, and the patient dies in 2 to 4 days. In extensive basilar infarction associated with deep comas, the patient seldom lives for more than a few days. Respiratory and urinary infection are constant dangers and once they begin, there is usually a rapid decline in the patient's conditions. His temperature rises. In the case of small infarcts, recovery may start within hours or a day or two and restoration may be complete. In cases of severe deficit, there may be no significant recovery whatsoever and after months of assiduous efforts at rehabilitation, the patient may remain bereft of speech with the upper extremity, still totally useless and the lower extremity serving only as an uncertain prop in attempting to walk. It is safer to say, the longer the delay before movement begins, the poorer the prognosis becomes. If recovery is not started in one or two weeks, the outlook is gloomy both for motor activity and speech and in general it may be said that whatever motor paralysis remains after 5 to 6 months will probably be permanent.

It is a fact to be discerned here that among the aforementioned signs and symptoms pertaining to prognosis as asserted in modern medicine, state of gambhira murcha (profound unconsciousness), extremely severe dhatu kshaya (depletion of supportive elements) involving the solitary area of the brain and puraanatva (chronicity) of disease - these three points correlate well with the opinions expressed in Ayurveda. Apart from this a person of Vata prakrti (constitution) who is born and grew up in Jangala desha (Arid province) and is also diseased, as also if the disease has commenced during Varsha rtu (Rainy season) and during old age, such samsargaja (coalescent) Pakshaghata may become formidable or is incurable.[Because of tulya prakrti (equivalent constitution), desha (geographical province) and kala (season)]. Similarly, Pakshaghata originating due to Vata and Pitta in a patient of Pitta prakrti (constitution) during the madhyama vaya (middle age) as well as in Sharad rtu (Autumn season) may become formidable or incurable. In the same patient Shudha Vataja (exclusively of Vata) Pakashaghata may become alpakrchra sadhya (marginally amenable). Shudha Vataja (exclusively due to Vata) Pakshaghata in a patient of Kapha prakrti (constitution) where the onset is in Vasanta rtu (Spring season) as also during childhood may become alpa krchra sadhya (marginally amenable) and Pakshaghata due to Vatakapha may become krchra sadhya (formidable) or asadhya (incurable). In this manner physician will have to decide through self-deliberation the prognosis of this disease based upon the tulya / atulya (equivalent / disparate) state of dosha (vitiator), prakrti (constitution), desha (province), kala (season), and vaya (age).The prognosis of this disease based on the equivalence of dosha (vitiator), desha (province), rtu (season), prakrti (constitution) and vaya (age) are indicated in the following table.

The knowledge pertaining to prognosis narrated so far from varied sources has been compiled in the following table.

Table Showing Sadhyasadhyata (Prognosis) of Pakshaghata

Number	Points to be Pondered	Sadhya (Curable)	Krchra Sadhya (Formidable)	Asadhya (Incurable)
1.	Dosha (Vitiator)	Vata kaphaja Vata pittaja	ShudhaVataja	
2.	Dhatu kshaya (Depletion of supportive tissues)	-----------------------	Dhatu kshaya due to common causes	Asrk kshayaja mamsa kshaya (Emaciation of flesh due to diminution ofblood)
3.	Roga nidana (Diagnosis of illness)			If exact diagnosis of illness has not been made.
4.	Chikitsa (Treatment)	-----------------------	-----------------------	If appropriate treatment hasnot been given
5.	Upadrava (supervenient afflictions)	Nirupadrava (Absence of supervenient afflictions)		Upadravayukta (Accompanied with supervenient afflictions)

6.	Adhistana(Abode)	-----------------------	---------------------	Gambhira stana stita (Grave Locus)
7.	Bala (Strength)	Sabala (strong)	Sabala (strong)	Durbala (weak)
8.	Vyadhi kala (chronicity)	Up to 5months	9 –12 months	More than one year
9.	Vaya (Age)	-----------------	Middle age	Childhood and old age
10.	Indriya stiti (Status of sensory organs)			Sparsha hani yukta (Accompanied with loss of tactility)
11.	Anushangika lakshanas (Other concomitant attributes)	-----------------------	----------------------	1. Change of colour in the aberrant extremities 2. Shota (oedema) 3. Kampa (tremors) 4. Adhmana (Tympanitis) 5.Gambiramurcha (Profound unconsciousness)

12.Classification Based on Tulya/atulya (Equivalent/Disparate) Dosha, Prakrti, Desha, Kala

Number	Dosha Vitiator	Prakrti Constitution	Desha Geogra–phical Province	Vaya Age	Kala Season	Sadhya Asadhya Prognosis
1.	Vata	Vata	Jangala Arid	Vrdhapya Old age	Varsha Rainy	Asadhya Incurable
2.	Vata	Vata	Anupa Humid Sadharana Nonspecific	Balya Childhood Madhyama Middle age	Sharath Autumn Vasanta Spring	Sadhya Curable
3.	Vatapitta	Vata Pitta Vatapitta	Jangala Arid	Madhyama Middle age	Varsha Rainy Sharath Autumn	Krchrasadhya Formidable
4.	Vatapitta	Kapha	Anupa Humid Sadarana Nonspecific	Balya Childhood	Vasanta Spring	Krchra sadhya Formidable
5.	Vatakapha	Kapha	Anupa Humid	Balya Childhood	Vasanta Spring	Asadya Incurable
6.	Vatakapha	Pitta	Sadharana Non-specific	Madhyama Middle age	Sharath Autumn	Susadhya Easily curable

It is left to the research scholars of Ayurveda to meticulously observe the prognostications mentioned above in the core texts of Ayurveda and clarify the karya karana(cause and effect) of roga samprapti (disease pathogenesis).

If the disease is found to be curable, after observing meticulously all the factors, the therapeutic sequence should be employed as enumerated in the classics.

Examination of the Patient

1) **Prashna Pareeksha (Examination Through Questions)–**

   a. **Food** – Is the patient habituated to consuming more of snigdha (unctuous) substances like oil, ghee, milk, curd, flesh, etc., or does he consume more of ruksha ahara (coarse food) that is excessively katu (pungent), tikta (bitter), kashaya (astringent), or does he consume more food that aggravates Vata such as potatoes, tur dal, brinjal, etc.? Does he always consume excessive cold food and drinks?

   b. **Pertaining to pastime**: Does he have a vrthi (profession) or vyavahara (enterprise) or vihara (pastime) that enhances sheeta guna (attributes of cold) or depletes bala (strength) and mamsa (flesh).

   c. **Pertaining to vichara (cerebration)**: Pertaining to shoka (grief) and krodha (anger) should be queried and discerned.

   d. **Pertaining to onset of illness:** Is the onset with murcha (unconsciousness)? Or is the onset insidious? Or is the onset sequential (slowly)?

e. **Pertaining to geographical area**: Questions essential to understand as to among the 3 types of geographical area such as Jangala (Arid) etc., in which geographical area the patient was born, grew up and became ill.

f. **Pertaining to time**: Age of the patient, in which season among Grishma (Summer) etc. the onslaught of the disease occurred? What is the duration of the illness (more than one year or not)?

g. **Pertaining to nidana (diagnosis) and chikitsa (treatment)**: Has it been shown to any other physician in the past, has treatment been carried out, if so, what are the treatments undertaken? (To understand whether diagnosis and treatment have been appropriately and punctually carried out)

h. **Pertaining to prodromal signs and symptoms (purva rupa)**: Shortly before onset of illness was there a headache etc.?

i. **Pertaining to other antecedent illnesses (purva vyadhi)**: was there purva vyadhi (antecedent illnesses) such as blood pressure, etc.?

This is the important information to be gathered.

2. **Darshana pareeksha (Visual examination)**: Patients gamana vidhana (gait) and pratyavartana (reflex) of janu (thighs), pada (feet) and udara (abdomen) should be specifically observed. Is there shosha (emaciation), shota (edema) or vaivarnya (discolouration) etc., present in the vikrta parshwa (aberrant extremities)? Is

the arm placed in a distinctive manner? Is there kriya hani (attenuated functions) of hand and feet (variety of movements), whether any mukhardha vikrti (aberrant facial half) is present, etc., should be understood through detailed visual examination.

3. **Sparshana pareeksha (Examination through palpation)**: Does the muscles on the vikrta parshwa (aberrant extremities) appear katina (hardened)? shitila (flaccid)? How is the grahana shakti (grasping power) of fingers of the hand? The status of sheetoshna stiti (warmth / coldness) of the skin, nadi gati (pulse rate), yati (rhythm), samhati (compactness), aakrti (form) etc., should be examined and noted.

4. **Anya (Others):** Whether sparsha jnana (tactile sensation) is normal or is aberrant? Examination pertaining to upadrava (supervenient afflictions) like Hrdroga (Heart disease), Gulma (Phantom tumours) and Visarpa (Herpes) should be carried out. Status of Raktachapa (Blood pressure) should be invariably noted.

5. **Rasayanika (Biochemical)** and other examinations:

   Whether shirshambu- tarpaka kapha (cerebro spinal fluid) is blood stained or clear, etc. and serum cholesterol level should be examined.

5. **Cerebral angiography :** It is better to carry out cerebral angiography to know Cerebral thrombosis, Embolism, etc.

1. *vayuhu katyashritaha saktni kandaramakshipet yada/ khanjastada bhavejjantuhu panguhu saktnordvayorvadhat / (Su.ni.1/77)*
2. *... "tatra sparshajnanamadhaha kaye cheshtopaghatascha" (Su.sha.6/26)*
3. *..."janmabala pravrtta ye maturapacharat pangu jatyandhaha" (Su.su 24/*
4. *"saktna urdva janghayaha "(Ma.ko, va vya ni59) "gulphadi vitapantam saktihi"(Dalhana su.ni.1/74)*
5. *"douhridavimananat kubjam khanjam..sutam janayanti" (S.sha 3/18)*
6. *"sarvanga rogam tadvaccha sarva kayashrite anile" (A. hr.ni.15/40)*
7. *"ekanga vikaramiti ekasminnange ya utpadyate sa ekangavikaram sa chatra vata janitaha" (Dalhana su su14/30_)*
8. *"vakribhavati vaktrardham"(Su.ni1/60)*
9. *"shareerardhamekam vayuhu prapadhyate/ ardhe tasmin mukhardheva kevale syatardatadam(Cha.chi28/38-42) 10... "bahvoho karma kshayakari' (Su.ni 1/75)*
11. *... "bahvoriti dvivachanam, samanyapekshaya,kadachit tasminchidbahou bhavati" (Dalhana su.ni 1/75)*

CHAPTER – 8

Chikitsa Prakarana
Treatise on Therapeutics

While treating this illness the following points should be mainly considered.

1. The sanga (blockage) that has arisen in the indriyadhistana-shiras (abode of the sense organs – head) should be resolved.

2. The "Mastulunga majja" [brain (marrow)] that is dushita (vitiated) should be purified.

3. Proper circulation of rasa/rakta (lymph/ blood) to the shiras (head) should be ascertained.

4. Appropriate sneha poshana (oleaginous nourishment) of Mastulunga (Brain), sira (arteries) and snayu (muscles) should be ascertained.

To accomplish the aforesaid objectives our ancestors have chronicled several lines of treatment. These will be described in systematic order later on.

Since Pakshaghata is a disease of Vata, all upakrama (therapeutic measures) ascribed for diseases of Vata will be beneficial in Pakshaghata also. However, since authors of manifold texts have specially referred to multifold lines of treatment, these may be recognized as specialized lines of treatment for Pakshaghata also.

Acoording to Drdabalacharya

1. Snehana (Unction)
2. Svedana (Diaphoresis)
3. Virechana (Laxation)

are the three specialized lines of treatment.

Svedanam sneha samyuktam pakshaghate virechanam (Cha. chi. 28 / 100).

These three itself have been reiterated in Ashtanga hrdaya and Ashtanga samgraha also.

Snehanam sneha samyuktam pakshaghate virechanam (A.hr.chi.21/44)

Snehanam sveda samyuktam pakshaghate virechanam (A.Sam. Chi. 21/44).

Some have inferred the above-mentioned core verses of Ashtanga hrdaya depicting snehana (unction) and sneha yukta virechana (oleaginous laxation), as specialized lines of treatment for Pakshaghata. This verse does not carry a reference to the performance of svedana (diaphoresis). Does it mean that as per Vagbhata's opinion svedana (diaphoresis) is not essential in Pakshaghata? Probably it is not so. Hence, in this context it appears appropriate to cognize snehadhara sveda (oleaginous cascade diaphoresis) by the word snehana. The meaning of the phraseology sneha samyukta virechana (oleaginous laxation) cropping up in the same verse has to be that in Pakshaghata sneha virechana (oleaginous laxation) should be administered. Meaning virechana (laxation) should be ordained through Eranda taila (castor oil), Tilvaka ghrta (ghee of Tilvaka), etc. However rather than the assertion that in Pakshaghata exclusively sneha samyukta virechana (oleaginous laxation) should be administered, it is preferable to assume that sneha samyukta virechana (oleaginous laxation) is superior to ruksha virechana (coarse laxation) through churna (pulverized powder).

According to Sushrutacharya the following are the specialized lines of treatment.

1. Snehana (Unction)
2. Svedana (Diaphoresis)
3. Mrdu samshodhana (Gentle purification)
4. Anuvasana (Oleaginous enema)
5. Astapana (Astringent enema)
6. Line of treatment indicated in Akshepa (convulsions)
7. Specially Mastishkya [External therapy to the head (a form of therapeutic pad to the head)]
8. Shirobasti (a type of external medicament to the head through cumulation of oil)

Tatra prageva sneha svedopapannam
mrduna shodhanena samshodhya anuvasya
astapya cha yata kalamakshepaka
vidhanenopachareth ;
vaisheshikaschatra mastishkyaha shirovasti (Su.chi.5/19)

Apart from this while narrating the qualities of some formulations of oils, etc. various texts have apprised as to how to make use of them. Based on this, indications are available on a few more lines of treatment – Karna purana (instillation of medicament into ear) or Nasya (instillation of medicament into the nose) etc. that can be employed in Pakshaghata. All these methods are shown concisely in the ensuing tables.

CHIKITSA TALIKA

Therapeutic Table

- 1. Nidana parivarjana (Eschewal of etiology)
  - Ahara Food
  - Vihara lifestyle
  - Vichara cerebration
- 2. Shodhana (Purification)
  - Purva karma Pre operative procedure
    - If essential Deepana (kindlers) Pachana (digestives)
    - Sneha pana (Oleaginous oral administration)
    - Abhyanga (unction)
    - Sveda (Diaphoresis)
  - Pradhana karma Cardinal procedure
    - Mrdu virechana (mild laxation)
    - Anuvasana (oleaginous enema)
    - Aastapana (astringent enema)
    - Nasya (Nasal instillation)
  - Paschath karma Ensuing procedure
    - Peyadi samsarjana or tarpana (conciliatory sequence with thin gruel etc. or nurture → Mrdu virechana; → Anuvasana)
- 3. Shamana (Palliation)

3. Shamana (Palliation)

- Bahihi parimarjana (External purification)
  - Karna Purana Instillation to ears
  - Shiro abhyanga Unction to the head
  - Shiraha Seka Fomentation to the head
  - Shirah pichu (oleaginous pad to the head)
  - Shiro basti (cumulation of oil on head)
  - Akshi tarpana (Nurture to eyes)
  - Viktrta parshva abhyanga Unction to the aberrant half
  - Sveda (Diaphoresis)
- Antaha parimarjana (Internal purification)
  - Snehapana Oleaginous oral administration
  - Kashaya Decoction
  - Kalka Pulp or paste
  - Churna Pulverized powder
  - Vati pills
  - Anya Others

All these cannot be started simultaneously. Such a beginning is not appropriate too. Hence in which sequence it should be started. Which of these have to be administered for what minimum number of days? And approximately how many days are required to complete one cycle of this line of treatment, etc. have been described in the ensuing pages.

Generally, if a patient of Pakshaghata is brought to a physician in a state of unconsciousness (early) he should be administered sadyo sanjna prabhodhana chikitsa (treatment that helps to restore consciousness immediately). For this pradhamana nasya (a form of nasal instillation where medicinal particles are blown into the nose) with pulverized Svaskutar ras or Murchantaka ras can be employed Or Avapeedaka nasya (where medication is squeezed in to the nose) – with lashuna kalka (garlic pulp) can be used. After the patient recovers from unconsciousness other lines of treatment should be systematically employed.

Initially to digest saamadosha (dosha vitiated by ama) it is better to administer any of the digestive medicines such as Panchakola churna (pulverized powder) or kashaya (decoction) at an appropriate dosage and duration until nirama lakshana (innocuous attributes) come into manifestation. Subsequently up to a maximum of 7 days krama vridhi snehapana (sequential ascending oleaginous oral administration) should be done or it should be administered till samyak snigdha lakshana (apt signs and symptoms of appropriate unctuous suffusion), come into manifestation. (No need to wait till seven days). During this period after the snehapana (oleaginous oral administration), based upon the sneha (unctuous substance), anupana such as hot water, yusha (broth), etc., as well as after digestion of the sneha (unctuous substance) light hot food, should be consumed. Foods that are madhura (sweet), sheeta (cold), guru (heavy) such as bananas, apples and grapes are contraindicated. Not only that, administration of any shamana oushadha (palliative medicine) is also unnecessary. Pathya krama (Congenial dietary sequence) such as drinking of hot water should be followed. Subsequent to manifestation of signs and symptoms of samyak snigdha lakshana (apt signs and symptoms of appropriate unctuous suffusion), sarvanga abhyanga (full body unction) should be carried out and svedana (diaphoresis) with bashpa (steam) or pinda (clod) should be given. Sneha dhara sveda (Diaphoresis through oil cascade) can be given. Where sneha dhara sveda (diaphoresis through oil cascade) is administered there is no need for separate abhyanga (unction). In this manner the sequence of snehana (unction) and svedana (diaphoresis) should be carried out for three days. During this period pathyahara (congenial diet) shown here afterwards should be given. After repetition of abhyanga (unction) and svedana (diaphoresis) again, virechana (laxation) should be given in the morning around 9 am. For virechana (laxation) Eranda taila (castor oil) 30-60ml should be given with hot milk or hot water as needed. The category of purification {(pravara (exalted), madhyama (moderate), avara (inferior)}following administration of this form of virechana (laxation) should be discerned and based on that ahara samsarjana krama (sequential conciliatory food) should be employed. This samsarjana krama (conciliatory sequence) can be started from the evening itself of the day virechana (laxation) is administered. During the period when this samsarjana (conciliatory procedure) is in progress Mashadi kwata (decoction of black gram) etc. 15-30ml or any of the appropriate shamanoushadha (palliative medicine) can be given from the list of shamanoushadha (palliative medicines) provided at the concluding part of this text. At this point of time, it is not necessary to give basti (enema) or snehadhara sveda (diaphoretic oleaginous cascade). However, shiro pichu (oleaginous head pad), karna purana (instillation of ears) and nasya (instillation of nose) can be administered. After completion of samsarjana krama (conciliatory sequence) and consumption of prakrta bhojana (normal food) is accomplished, on the ninth day from the day of virechana (laxation) basti krama (sequential enema) should be started.Niruhabasti (enema with decoction) and appropriate sneha basti (oleaginous enema) with Vata hara kwata (decoctions that eliminate Vata) narrated here afterwards, should be given in the form of Karma basti (functional enema), Kala basti (chronological enema) or Yoga basti (composite enema) as required.The list of oils useful in anuvasana basti (oleaginous enema) has been given towards the end of this book. Anyone of them can be employed. The same kwata (decoction) of the substances that are indicated as suitable for anuvasana basti (oleaginous enema) can be used for niruha basti (enema with decoction). After the completion of the basti chikitsa (therapeutic enema) rasa samsarjana krama (sequential conciliatory procedure based on savoury) should be followed.

During the course of basti krama (sequential enema)

shamanoushadha (palliative medication) in the form of Ekanga veer rasa, etc. [with the exception of sneha (unctuous)] can be given. **Not only that from the day of commencement of basti itself, shirobasti (a form of external cumulative oil therapy to the head) or mastishkya (a form of external therapy to the brain), karna purana (instillation of ears), kayaseka (fomentation to the body) can be carried out as needed.** After completion of basti krama (sequential enema), exclusively snehadhara sveda (oleaginous steam cascade diaphoresis) and shamanoushada (palliative medications) -- (as internal administration) should be given for one week (minimum). During this period nasya should be administered with Mahamasha taila or any other suitable oil. In this manner after administration of shamanoushadha (palliative medicines) for 1 week (more or less), again in the same aforementioned sequence snehapana (oleaginous oral administration), virechana (laxation) and basti (enema) should be administered. In this way in the second or subsequent cycle, it is sufficient if sadya snehapana (proximate oleaginous oral admiistration) is carried out prior to virechana (laxation). In this way repeated treatment should be carried out sequentially in the form of shodhana (purification) and shamana (palliation) for a duration of 3-4 months.

"Tatra prageva snehasvedopapannam mrduna shodhanena samshodhyanuvasyacha yatakalamakshepaka vidhanena upachareth, salvanamupahanarte, balatailamanuvasanarte, evam atandritaha treen chaturo va masan kriyapathamupaseveta"

Su.sam.chi.5/19

Chronological Table for Treatment of Pakshaghata - Up To Date Description

Chikitsa Krama **Mode of Treatment**	**Krura Kosta** **Costic Bowel**	**Madhyama Kosta** **Moderate Bowel**	**Mrdu Kosta** **Delicate Bowel**
Samapachana and agnideepana (Digestion of the noxious element and enkindle)	Anirdhista kala Indefinite period	Anirdhista kala Indefinite period	Anirdhista kala Indefinite period
Snehapana (Oleaginous oral administration)	For a duration of seven days subsequent to manifestation of attributes of nirama dosha (innocuous dosha)	For a duration of five days subsequent to manifestation of attributesof nirama dosha (innocuous dosha)	For a duration of three days subsequent to manifestation of attributes of nirama dosha (innocuous dosha)
Rest preparatory to Virechana	From8th day to 10th day [during these three days whole body abhyanga (unction) and sveda (diaphoresis) should be done and snigdhoshna ahara (unctuous hot food) should be given].	From 6th day to 8$^{th\ day}$ [during these three days whole body abhyanga (unction) and sveda (diaphoresis) should be done and snigdhoshna ahara (unctuous hot food) should be given]	From 4th day to 6$^{th\ day}$ [during these three days whole body abhyanga (unction) and sveda (diaphoresis) should be done and snigdhoshna ahara (unctuous hot food) should be given]
Virechana	11th day	9th day	7th day

3. Samsarjana (Pacification)

Krura koshta
(Costive Bowel)

DAY	Pravara Shudhi Exalted Purity	Madhyama Shudhi Moderate Purity	Avara Shudhi Inferior Purity
11E	Peya Thin gruel	Peya Thin gruel	Peya Thin gruel
12M	Peya Thin gruel	Peya Thin gruel	Vilepi Moderately thick gruel
12E	Peya thin gruel	Vilepi Moderately thick gruel	Akrta yusha or Akrta mamsa (Unseasoned thin greengram soup or unseasoned mutton soup)
13M	Vilepi Moderately thick gruel	Vilepi Moderately thick gruel	Krta yusha or Krta mamsa rasa (Seasoned thin greengram soup or seasoned mutton soup)
13E	Vilepi Moderately thick gruel	Akrta yusha or Akrta mamsa rasa (Unseasoned thin greengram soup or unseasoned mutton soup)	Normal Diet
14M	Vilepi Moderately thick gruel	Akrta yusha or Akrta mamsa rasa (Unseasoned thin greengram soup or unseasoned mutton soup)	Normal diet

DAY	Pravara Shudhi Exalted Purity	Madhyama Shudhi Moderate Purity	Avara Shudhi Inferior Purity
14E	Akrta yusha or Akrta mamsa rasa (Unseasoned thin greengram soup or unseasoned mutton soup)	Krta yusha or Krta mamsa rasa (Seasoned thin greengram soup or seasoned mutton soup)	Normal diet
15M	Akrta yusha or Akrta mamsa (Unseasoned thin greengram soup or unseasoned mutton soup)	Krta yusha or Krta mamsa rasa (Seasoned thin greengram soup or seasoned mutton soup)	Normal diet
15E	Akrta yusha or Akrta mamsa rasa (Unseasoned thin greengram soup or unseasoned mutton soup)	Normal diet	Normal diet
16M	Krta yusha or Krta mamsa rasa (Seasoned thin greengram soup or seasoned mutton soup)	Normal diet	Normal diet

DAY	Pravara Shudhi Exalted Purity	Madhyama Shudhi Moderate Purity	Avara Shudhi Inferior Purity
16E	Krta yusha or Krta mamsa rasa (Seasoned thin greengram soup or seasoned mutton spoup)	Normal diet	Normal diet
17M	Krta yusha or Krta mamsa rasa (Seasoned thin greengram soup or seasoned mutton soup)	Normal diet	Normal diet
17E	Normal diet	Normal diet	Normal diet

Madhyama Koshta (Moderate Bowel)

Day	Pravara Shudhi (Exalted Purity)	Madhyama Shudhi (Moderate Purity)	Avara Shudhi (Inferior Purity)
9E	Peya Thin gruel	Peya Thin gruel	Peya Thin gruel
10M	Peya Thin gruel	Peya Thin gruel	Vilepi Moderately thick gruel

Day	Pravara Shudhi (Exalted Purity)	Madhyama Shudhi (Moderate Purity)	Avara Shudhi (Inferior Purity)
10E	Peya Thin gruel	Vilepi Moderately thick gruel	Akrta yusha or Akrta mamsa rasa Unseasoned thin greengram soup or Unseasoned mutton soup
11M	Vilepi Moderately thick gruel	Vilepi Moderately thick gruel	Krta yusha or Krta mamsa rasa Seasoned thin greengram soup or Seasoned mutton soup
11E	Vilepi Moderately thick gruel	Akrta yusha or Akrta mamsa rasa Unseasoned thin greengram soup or Unseasoned as mutton soup	Normal diet
12M	Vilepi Moderately thick gruel	Akrta yusha or Akrta mamsa rasa Unseasoned thin greengram soup or Unseasoned mutton soup	Normal diet
12E	Akrta yusha or Akrta mamsa rasa Unseasoned thin greengram soup or Unseasoned mutton soup	Krta yusha or Krta mamsa rasa Seasoned thin greengramsoup or Seasoned mutton soup	Normal diet

Day	Pravara Shudhi (Exalted Purity)	Madhyama Shudhi (Moderate Purity)	Avara Shudhi (Inferior Purity)
13M	Akrta yusha or Akrta mamsa rasa Unseasoned thin greengram soup or unseasoned mutton soup	Krta yusha or Krta mamsa rasa Seasoned thin greengram soup or seasoned mutton soup	Normal diet
13E	Akrta yusha or Akrta mamsa rasa Unseasoned thin greengram soup or Unseasoned mutton soup	Normal diet	Normal diet
14M	Krta yusha or Krta mamsa rasa Seasoned thin greengram soup or Seasoned mutton soup	Normal diet	Normal diet
14E	Krta yusha or Krta mamsa rasa Seasoned thin greengram soup or Seasoned mutton soup	Normal diet	Normal diet
15M	Krta yusha or Krta mamsa rasa Seasoned thin greengram soup or Seasoned mutton soup	Normal diet	Normal diet
15E	Normal diet	Normal diet	Normal diet

Mrdu Koshta
(Delicate Bowel)

Day	Pravara Shudhi (Exalted Purity)	Madhyama Shudhi (Moderate Purity)	Avara Shudhi (Inferior Purity)
7E	Peya thin gruel	Peya thin gruel	Peya thin gruel
8M	Peya thin gruel	Peya thin gruel	Vilepi Moderately thick gruel
8E	Peya thin gruel	Vilepi Moderately thick gruel	Akrta yusha or Akrta mamsa rasa Unseasoned thin greengram soup or Unseasoned mutton soup
9M	Vilepi Moderately thick gruel	Vilepi Moderately thick gruel	Krta yusha or Krta mamsa Seasoned thin greengram soup or seasoned mutton soup
9E	Vilepi Moderately thick gruel	Akrta yusha or Akrta mamsa rasa Unseasoned thin greengram soup or Unseasoned mutton soup	Normal diet
10M	Vilepi Moderately thick gruel	Akrta yusha or Akrta mamsa rasa Unseasoned thin greengram soup or Unseasoned mutton soup	Normal diet

Day	Pravara Shudhi (Exalted Purity)	Madhyama Shudhi (Moderate Purity)	Avara Shudhi (Inferior Purity)
10E	Akrta yusha or Akrta mamsa rasa Unseasoned thin greengram soup or Unseasoned mutton soup	Krta yusha or Krta mamsa rasa (Seasoned thin greengram soup or Seasoned mutton soup)	Normal diet
11M	Akrta yusha or Akrta mamsa rasa Unseasoned thin greengram soup or Unseasoned mutton soup	Krta yusha or Krta mamsa rasa (Seasoned thin greengram soup or seasoned mutton soup)	Normal diet
11E	Akrta yusha or Akrta mamsa rasa Unseasoned thin greengram soup or Unseasoned mutton soup	Normal diet	Normal diet
12M	Krta yusha or Krta mamsa rasa Seasoned thin greengram soup or seasoned mutton soup	Normal diet	Normal diet

Day	Pravara Shudhi (Exalted Purity)	Madhyama Shudhi (Moderate Purity)	Avara Shudhi (Inferior Purity)
12E	Krta yusha or Krta mamsa rasa Seasoned thin greengram soup or seasoned mutton soup	Normal diet	Normal diet
13M	Krta yusha or Krta mamsa rasa Seasoned thin greengram soup or seasoned mutton soup	Normal diet	Normal diet
13E	Normal diet	Normal diet	Normal diet

Basti Chikitsa – Therapeutic Enema

DAY	Karma basti (Operative enema)	Kala basti (Chrono-logical enema)	Yoga basti (Composite enema)	DAY	Karma basti (Operative Enema)	Kala basti (Chrono-logical enema)	Yoga basti (Composite œnema)	DAY	Karma basti (Operative enema)	Kala basti (Chrono-logical enema)	Yoga basti (Composite enema)
19	Anuvasana	Anuvasana	Anuvasana	17	Anuvasana	Anuvasana	Anuvasana	15	Anuvasana	Anuvasana	Anuvasana
20	Niruha	Niruha	Niruha	18	Niruha	Niruha	Niruha	16	Niruha	Niruha	Niruha
21	Anuvasana	Anuvasana	Anuvasana	19	Anuvasan	Anuvasana	Anuvasana	17	Anuvasana	Anuvasana	Anuvasana
22	Niruha	Niruha	Niruha	20	Niruha	Niruha	Niruha	18	Niruha	Niruha	Niruha
23	Anuvasana	Anuvasana	Anuvasana	21	Anuvasana	Anuvasana	Anuvasana	19	Anuvasana	Anuvasana	Anuvasana
24	Niruha	Niruha	Niruha	22	Niruha	Niruha	Niruha	20	Niruha	Niruha	Niruha
25	Anuvasana	Anuvasana	Anuvasana	23	Anuvasana	Anuvasana	Anuvasana	21	Anuvasana	Anuvasana	Anuvasana
26	Niruha	Niruha	Anuvasana	24	Niruha	Niruha	Anuvasana	22	Niruha	Niruha	Anuvasana
27	Anuvasana	Anuvasana	---	25	Anuvasana	Anuvasana	-----	23	Anuvasana	Anuvasana	---------
28	Niruha	Niruha	---	26	Niruha	Niruha	--------	24	Niruha	Niruha	----------
29	Anuvasana	Anuvasana	---	27	Anuvasana	Anuvasana	---	25	Anuvasana	Anuvasana	--------
30	Niruha	Niruha	---	28	Niruha	Niruha	---	26	Niruha	Niruha	--------
31	Anuvasana	Anuvasana	---	29	Anuvasana	Anuvasana	---	27	Anuvasana	Anuvasana	---
32	Niruha	Anuvasana	---	30	Niruha	Anuvasana	---	28	Niruha	Anuvasana	---
33	Anuvasana	Anuvasana	---	31	Anuvasana	Anuvasana	---	29	Anuvasana	Anuvasana	---

DAY	Karma basti (Operative enema)	Kala basti (Chrono-logical enema)	Yoga basti (Composite enema)	DAY	Karma basti (Operative Enema)	Kala basti (Chrono-logical enema)	Yoga basti (Composite enema)	DAY	Karma basti (Operative enema)	Kala basti (Chrono-logical enema)	Yoga basti (Composite enema)
34	Niruha	Anuvasana	---	**32**	Niruha	Anuvasana	---	**30**	Niruha	Anuvasana	---
35	Anuvasana	------	---	33	Anuvasana	---	---	31	Anuvasana	---	---
36	Niruha	---	---	**34**	Niruha	---	---	**32**	Niruha	---	---
37	Anuvasana	---	---	**35**	Anuvasana	---	---	**33**	Anuvasana	---	---
38	Niruha	---	---	**36**	Niruha	---	---	**34**	Niruha	---	---
39	Anuvasana	---	---	**37**	Anuvasana	---	---	**35**	Anuvasana	---	---
40	Niruha	---	---	**38**	Niruha	---	---	**36**	Niruha	---	---
41	Anuvasana	---	---	**39**	Anuvasana	---	---	**37**	Anuvasana	---	---
42	Niruha	---	---	**40**	Niruha	---	---	**38**	Niruha	---	---
43	Anuvasana	---	---	**41**	Anuvasana	---	---	**39**	Anuvasana	---	---
44	Anuvasana	---	---	**42**	Anuvasana	---	---	**40**	Anuvasana	---	---
45	Anuvasana	---	---	**43**	Anuvasana	---	---	**41**	Anuvasana	---	---
46	Anuvasana	---	---	**44**	Anuvasana	---	---	**42**	Anuvasana	---	---
47	Anuvasana	---	---	**45**	Anuvasana	---	---	**43**	Anuvasana	---	---
48	Anuvasana	---	---	**46**	Anuvasana	---	---	**44**	Anuvasana	---	---

Rasa Samsarjana
(Conciliation by Savoury)

49 **M**	Madhura Sweet Amla Sour	Madhura Sweet Amla Sour	Madhura Sweet Amla Sour	**47** **M**	Madhura Sweet Amla Sour	Madhura Sweet Amla Sour	Madhura Sweet Amla Sour	**45** **M**	Madhura Sweet Amla Sour	Madhura Sweet Amla Sour	Madhura Sweet Amla Sour
49 **E**	Madhura Sweet Amla Sour	Madhura Sweet Amla Sour	Amla Sour Lavana Salty	**47** **E**	Madhura Sweet Amla Sour	Madhura Sweet Amla Sour	Amla Sour Lavana Salty	**45** **E**	Madhura Sweet Amla Sour	Madhura Sweet Amla Sour	Amla Sour Lavana Salty
50 **M**	Madhura Sweet Amla Sour	Amla Sour Lavana Salty	Madhura Sweet Tikta Bitter	**48** **M**	Madhura Sweet Amla Sour	Amla Sour Lavana Salty	Madhura Sweet Tikta Bitter	**46** **M**	Madhura Sweet Amla Sour	Amla Sour Lavana Salty	Madhura Sweet Tikta Bitter
50 **E**	Amla Sour Lavana Salty	Amla Sour Lavana Salty	Katu Pungent Kashaya Astringent	**48** **E**	Amla Sour Lavana Salty	Amla Sour Lavana Salty	Katu Pungent Kashaya Astringent	**46** **E**	Amla Sour Lavana Salty	Amla Sour Lavana Salty	Katu Pungent Kashaya Astringent
51 **M**	Amla Sour Lavana Salty	Madhura Sweet Tikta Bitter	Prakrta Bhojana Normal food	**49** **M**	Amla Sour Lavana Salty	Madhura Sweet Tikta Bitter	Prakrta Bhojana Normal food	**47** **M**	Amla Sour Lavana Salty	Madhura Sweet Tikta Bitter	Prakrta Bhojana Normal food

51 **E**	Amla Sour Lavana Salty	Madhura Sweet Tikta Bitter	Prakrta Bhojana Normal food	**49** **E**	Amla Sour Lavana Salty	Madhura Sweet Tikta Bitter	Prakrta Bhojana Normal food	**47** **E**	Amla Sour Lavana Salty	Madhura Sweet Tikta Bitter	Prakrta Bhojana Normal food
52 **M**	Madhura Sweet Tikta Bitter	Katu Pungent Kashaya Astringent	Prakrta Bhojana Normal Food	**50** **M**	Madhura Sweet Tikta Bitter	Katu Pungent Kashaya Astringent	Prakrta Bhojana Normal Food	**48** **M**	Madhura Sweet Tikta Bitter	Katu Pungent Kashaya Astringent	Prakrta Bhojana Normal Food
52 **E**	Madhura Sweet Tikta Bitter	Katu Pungent Kashaya Astringent	Prakrta Bhojana Normal food	**50** **E**	Madhura Sweet Tikta Bitter	Katu Pungent Kashaya Astringent	Prakrta Bhojana Normal food	**48** **E**	Madhura Sweet Tikta Bitter	Katu Pungent Kashaya Astringent	Prakrta Bhojana Normal food
53 **M**	Madhura Sweet Tikta Bitter	Prakrta Bhojana Normal food	Prakrta Bhojana Normal food	**51** **M**	Madhura Sweet Tikta Bitter	Prakrta Bhojana Normal food	Prakrta Bhojana Normal food	**49** **M**	Madhura Sweet Tikta Bitter	Prakrta Bhojana Normal food	Prakrta Bhojana Normal food
53 **E**	Katu Pungent Kashaya Astringent	Prakrta Bhojana Normal food	Prakrta Bhojana Normal food	**51** **E**	Katu Pungent Kashaya Astringent	Prakrta Bhojana Normal food	Prakrta Bhojana Normal food	**49** **E**	Katu Pungent Kashaya Astringent	Prakrta Bhojana Normal food	Prakrta Bhojana Normal food

54 M	Katu Pungent Kashaya Astringent	Prakrta Bhojana Normal food	Prakrta Bhojana Normal food	**52 M**	Katu Pungent Kashaya Astringent	Prakrta Bhojana Normal food	Prakrta Bhojana Normal food	**50 M**	Katu Pungent Kashaya Astringent	Prakrta Bhojana Normal food	Prakrta Bhojana Normal food
54 E	Katu Pungent Kashaya Astringent	Prakrta Bhojana Normal food	Prakrta Bhojana Normal food	**52 E**	Katu Pungent Kashaya Astringent	Prakrta Bhojana Normal food	Prakrta Bhojana Normal food	**50 E**	Katu Pungent Kashaya Astringent	Prakrta Bhojana Normal food	Prakrta Bhojana Normal food
55 M	Prakrta Bhojana Normal food	Prakrta Bhojana Normal food	Prakrta Bhojana Normal food	**53 M**	Prakrta Bhojana Normal food	Prakrta Bhojana Normal food	Prakrta Bhojana Normal food	**51 M**	Prakrta Bhojana Normal food	Prakrta Bhojana Normal food	Prakrta Bhojana Normal food

After the basti chikitsa (therapeutic enema) rasa samsarjana krama (sequential conciliation by savoury) should be followed. This does not mean that only the specific rasa (savoury) should be administered. On the other hand, it should be understood that the above rasa (savoury) should be predominantly added on the respective days in the odana (porridge), and other food consumed by the patient.

After completion of one course of samshodhana (purification) as per aforementioned procedure for a duration of one week or slightly more Shiropichu (oleaginous cotton pad to the head), Karnapurana (instillation of ear), Nasya (instillation of nose), Snehadhara sveda (oleaginous cascade diaphoresis) and Shamanoushdha (palliative medications) should be followed along with pathya ahara (congenial diet) and vihara (congenial activities). After this if there is requirement of virechana (laxation) and basti (enema) again, virechana (laxation) should be given with preceding sadyaha snehana [proximate (immediate) oleaginous oral administration] and then after undergoing samsarjana krama (conciliatory sequence), basti (enema) should be administered as in the previous sequence.

Anyone can feel that if the aforementioned line of treatment is sequentially followed the total duration of treatment and its cost will be beyond the reach of a financially weak patient of our country. This is the reality. Moreover, Pakshaghata always do not happen to financially affluent people. It can happen to a poor patient. When this disease happens to a poor person classical line of treatment enumerated in ayurveda becomes only a day dream. Hence a situation may arise to plan a line of treatment at a lower cost to enable treatment of the illness. In such situations even though the total duration of treatment cannot be shortened, from the standpoint of financial expenditure, a line of treatment that can be employed with slightly less expenses can be commissioned as follows -

1. Sadyaha sneha [proximate (immediate) oleaginous oral administration] – Ghrita (ghee) + Lavana (salt) or Tila taila (sesame oil) + Lavana (salt) – 1st day

2. Abhyanga (unction) - (with suitable oil), Sveda (diaphoresis) (hot water bath), Laghu, Ushna, Snigdha ahara (light hot unctuous food) - 2nd day till 4th day

3. Virechana (laxation) – with Erand taila (castor oil) – on 5th day

4. Samsarjana krama (Conciliatory sequence) and employment of shamanoushadha (palliative medicine) from the evening of 5th day till maximum of 11th day

5. Prakrta bhojana (normal diet) – from 7th or 11th day

a. Nasya (nasal instillation) from the same day using Mahamasha taila

b. Ekanga veer rasa for one month

c. Shiro abhyanga (Unction of the head) – Abhyanga (unction) of the vikrta parshwa (aberrant side) and hot water bath - every day - for one month.

6. Commence second cycle of Sadhyaha sneha [proximate (immediate) oleaginous oral administration] again- in this manner treatment is essential for maximum of four months.

To further simplify this treatment, when necessary, at least following version should be followed:

(a) Abhyanga (unction) with Tila taila (sesame oil) (head to toe)

(b) Ushnodaka snana (hot water bath) (head to toe)

(c) Shiro pichu (oleaginous cotton pad to head) with Vatahara taila

(d) Mrdu virechana (mild laxation) using Haritaki churna (pulverized Haritaki)

(e) Mashadi or Rasnadi or Mahamanjishtadi decoction should be consumed with pathya ahara (congenial diet)- about 60ml of decoction - twice daily after food – for a duration of 2 months to maximum 4 months.

It would have been possible for us to provide financially very low-cost treatment if we did have the knowledge of applied aspects of agni karma (branding) as per the injunction in Basavarajiya "pakshayoho daheth" .(Agnikarma should be carried out on the vikrta parshwa (aberrant flank) in Pakshaghata). It is our misfortune that the flow of knowledge has become obliterated now. It appears that procedure for doing Agni karma (branding) in Pakshaghata is no more in existence in any corner of the country. For our research scholars Agni karma in Pakshaghata may constitute a worthy challenge.

Patient should be admitted as an in-patient and treated, from the standpoint of providing appropriate treatment as well as to ensure implementation of the aforementioned line of treatment. Due to inevitable circumstances if the patient cannot be admitted and treatment is to be the advised to be taken at his own residence following prescription can be given from the outpatient department.

1. Ekanga veera rasa - 150mg with honey before food thrice daily

2. Mahamashadi kwatha - 50ml thrice daily along with item no.1

3. Brihath Chagaladi ghrita- 20ml along with food twice daily or with milk twice daily.

4. Mahamasha taila – Shiro picchu (oleaginous cotton pad to head) for minimum 30minutes.

5. Abhyanga (unction) and snana (bath) – Abhyanga (unction) with Mahamasha or Vishatinduka taila followed by a hot water bath in the morning.

6. Nasya (nasal instillation) with Mahamasha taila – during evening.

Suitable pills, oil, etc. shamanoushadi (palliative medicine) mentioned here-after can be employed in the aforementioned manner.

Mode of Action of the Cardinal Line of Treatment Described So Far: -

1. **Shirobasti (Cumulative Medicament on Head)** – Medicated oil used in shirobasti predominantly possesses the properties of Ushna (torridity) and Snigdha (unctuosity). "Brajaka pitta" located in the skin gets stimulated because of the attribute of Ushna (torridity). As a result of this, Sneha

guna (attribute of unctuosity) of the oil and Veerya (potency) of medicines present in the oil are enabled entry through the skin into the circulation of rasa (plasma) and rakta (blood) (Su.sam.su). The Sneha (unctuosity) and Veerya (potency) of medicines so absorbed, after appropriate paka (refinement) through dhatvagni (metabolism) not only nourishes the Mastulunga majja (Brain matter) but the Veerya (potency) and Ushnata (torridity) present in the absorbed sneha (unctuosity) helps in dissolving the sangha (occlusion) present in the brain (dissolution of obstructive material). The substance causing the occlusion thus dissolved, enters rasa (plasma) and rakta (blood) and ultimately ends up in the koshta (visceral cavity). The substance causing the sangha (occlusion), thus reaching the koshta (visceral cavity) is thrown out through virechana (laxation). Concisely stated, this line of treatment results in the removal of the occlusion present in the Mastulunga (brain) which is indriyadhistana (abode of sensory organs) as well as causes nourishment of brain. The process of circulation of blood towards the brain is enhanced through the Ushna guna of sneha (attribute of torridity present in the unctuous) and nourishment of Mastishka (brain) occurs.

2. **Shiro abhyanga-seka-pichu (Unction - fomentation – oleaginous clod to the head)** - same activities described above occur to lesser extent.

3. **Nasya (Nasal Instillation)** - Due to teekshna (fiery) Avapidaka nasya [a form of nasya (nasal instillation) where medicament is squeezed in to the nose] with Lashuna kalka (pulp of garlic) the sangha (occlusion) confined to the

head is eliminated and Mastulunga (brain) is redeemed. In this context Sushrutacharya has espoused the mandatory use of Avapidaka nasya for shiraha shudhi (to purify the cephalum). Here it is appropriate to understand the word shudhi (purify) as removal of existing occlusion and ensuing proper circulation of blood. Meaning due to this the status of rakta poshanabhava (ischemic condition) of the brain becomes redeemed.

Nasya (Nasal instillation) with oil such as Mahamasha taila has twofold action.

Firstly, the attributes of Mastulunga majja (brain matter) gets enhanced (nourished) through the Snigdha - Guru guna (attributes of unctuosity and heaviness) of the oil. Secondly due to the Ushna and Kleda (attributes of torridity and moisture), the occlusive substance becomes dissolved and the sanga (occlusion) is eliminated and ensures that blood circulation is properly established.

4. **Karna purana (Instillation of Ears) and Akshi tarpana (Nurture of the Eyes)** - These two perform more or less the aforementioned actions.

5. **Abhyanga and Sveda (Unction and Diaphoresis)** – Brajaka Pitta that has skin as its abode gets roused through abhyanga (unction), and svedana (diaphoresis) (because of increased circulation of blood within the skin). The roused Brajaka Pitta aids in absorption of the veerya (potency) of the medicated oil employed in abhyanga (unction). The snehamsha (unctuosity) is absorbed to a small extent. The portion of snehamsha (unctuousness) thus absorbed enhances

the sneha bhava (unctuous facet) in the stanika sira (regional arteries) and snayu (muscles) and diminishes the sira snayu shosha lakshana (signs and symptoms of arterial and muscular emaciation). Because of this hands and legs of the vikrta parshwa (aberrant flank) gains strength. The svedana (diaphoresis) given after abhyanga (unction) enhances the circulation of blood and digests the snehamsha (unctuosity) absorbed through the skin aiding in deha satmikarana (systemic assimilation). These two actions not only perform regionally in the afore-mentioned manner but also dissolves the sangakaraka padarta (occluded substance) present in the head as well as performs the act of bringing this dissolved dushita padarta (vitiated substance) to the koshta (visceral cavity) through circulation of blood. Such dushita padarta (vitiated substance) entering the koshta (visceral cavity) is eliminated through virechana (laxation) or astapana basti (astringent enema).

Snehadhara Sveda – Pizhichil (Oleaginous Cascade diaphoresis) also does the same work of sneha – sveda (unction and diaphoresis) narrated above. Chakradutta (in the text) has advised employment of parishechana (sprinkling). It can be said that snehadhara sveda (oleaginous cascade diaphoresis) is an altered form of this parishechana (sprinkling).

6. **Avagahana (Immersion)** - Avagahana (immersion) in reality is a form of svedana (diaphoresis). However, the author of Bhaishajya ratnavali has indicated that taila droni avagahana (tub bath in medicated oil) should be carried out. Looking at this it appears that this procedure has been

advocated to derive the benefits of both snehana (unction) and svedana (diaphoresis) collectively. It appears there is no other intention other than this. The same Bhaishajya ratnavali has advocated 'Kanjika dronyavagahana' (immersion in a tub filled with fermented rice gruel) for a patient of Pakshaghata. The Kanjika (fermented rice gruel) that has been advocated for use here dominates in attributes of Ushna (torridity), Teekshna (fiery) and Amla (sour). The Amla rasa (Savoury of sourness) alleviates Vata. The attributes of Ushna (torridity) and Teekshna (fieriness) also alleviates Vata. Because of its attributes of Ushna (torridity) and Teekshna (fieriness) Kanjika enhances localized blood circulation and is competent in strengthening the sira (arteries) and snayu (muscles) present there. Hence it can be said that this is an appropriate procedure.

7. Virechana (Laxation) - According to Sushrutacharya mrdu samshodhana (gentle purification) should be employed in Pakshaghata. Customarily samshodhana (purification) connotes both vamana (emesis) and virechana (laxation). A question naturally arises as to whether, in Pakshaghata (Vatavyadhi), vamana (emesis) is appropriate. Commentator Dalhana also do not provide any clarification in this regard. Yet, since this is a disease of Vata it can be said that vamana (emesis) is not very appropriate. This resolution is supported by a clear directive in Charaka samhita and Ashtanga sangraha, wherein it is stated that in the aforementioned circumstance virechana (laxation) should be employed. Once it is decided that virechana (laxation) is appropriate, an uncertainty may arise as to whether mrdu virechana (gentle laxation) should be employed or as stated in Bhaishajya ratnavali teekshna virechana (drastic purgation) should be employed. Keeping in mind the patient's bala (strength) vayaha (age) and dushti teevrta (severity of defilement) decision has to be arrived at as to which one of these two, mrdu or teekshna virechana (gentle or drastic purgation) has to be carried out.

There is a good deal of description on the mode of action of this in many post-graduate dissertations. Broadly mode of action can be narrated in the following manner.

Virechana (laxation) mainly acts on Pittadhara kala (mucoid epithelium that sustains pitta) [Based on relationship between Pitta and virechana (laxation)]. Pittadhara kala has been regarded as Majjadhara kala [mucoid epithelium that sustains Majja (marrow)] also. Clarification has been provided in Sushruta samhita kalpa stana apropos visha vega (toxic celerity) that Pittadhara kala (mucoid epithelium that sustains pitta) itself should be understood as Majjadhara kala (marrow epithelium) (Dalhana- Sushruta.sam. kalpa 4/ 40). Probably this statement may have been made because there is no specific distinction between the rachana (anatomy) and kriya (physiological function) of these two. It can be presumed that all those that operate on Pittadhara kala (mucoid epithelium sustaining pitta) also exert similar prabhava (spell) on Majjadhara kala (marrow epithelium) also because of the sadharmya (homogeneity) between these two. Majjadhara kala (marrow epithelium) will be present wherever there is Majjadhatu (bone marrow). It has already been narrated in relation to samprapti (pathogenesis) of

Pakshaghata that there will be dushti (vitiation) of Majja (marrow) present in the Mastulunga (brain matter). Hence it can be said that the veerya (potency) of the virechaka oushadha (laxative drugs) acting on the Mastulunga majja (marrow of the brain), through the Majjadhara kala (marrow epithelium) throws out the Majja mala (defilement of the marrow) through the purisha (faeces).

The Majja mala (defilement of the marrow) has been explained as **"majnaha snehokshi vit tvacham"** - meaning vit sneha (unctuosity of faeces) is known as Majja mala (defilement of the marrow). In this manner since the Majja mala (defilement of majja) moves out in the form of purisha (unctuosity of the faeces) through virechana (laxation), Mastulunga majja (marrow of the brain) becomes purified.

This can be pictured briefly in the following manner.

Consumption of Virechaka Dravya (Laxative)

↓

(Its action on pittadhara kala (on mucoid epithelium of intestines)

↓

(Its action on majjadhara kala (marrow epithelium)

↓

{Joins Mastulunga majja (marrow of the brain)}

↓

{Segregates majja mala (purisha snehamsha) [defilement of the marrow]

↓

Purisha snehamsha (Unctuosity of faeces) reaches pittadharakala (Mucoid epithelium of intestines) through blood

↓

Purisha snehamsha (Unctuosity of faeces) is enhanced through this snehamsha (unctuosity)

↓

Snehamsha (majja mala) [defilement of the marrow] moves out along with faeces

↓

Mastulunga majja (marrow of the brain) is purified. Sanga (obstruction) in the Mastulunga (brain) is eliminated.

↓

Vata Shamana (Palliation of Vata)

It has been said that virechana (laxation) is the best form of shodhana (purification) for Pitta dosha. It can also be said that this is useful when Pakshaghata has samsarga (conjunction) of Pitta. Virechana (laxation) does not contravene Kapha dosha. Hence this can be employed even where there is anubandha (concomitance) of Kapha dosha. The benefits of virechana (laxation) in Pakshaghata can be endorsed from a different viewpoint also. There will be sira dushti (vitiation of arteries) [shosha - attenuation] in Pakshaghata. Sira (arteries) are upadhatu (ancillary supportive element) of blood. Virechana (laxation) acts on raktavaha srothas (blood vessels) also. It can be said that this helps in the elimination of sanga (blockages) present in it, thereby enabling adequate blood supply to the sira (arteries) and aids them in getting strengthened.

8. Basti (Enema)

a. Anuvasana Basti (Oleaginous Enema) – The prime ingredient of anuvasana basti (oleaginous enema) in Pakshaghata is taila (oil). Because of the Snigdha guna(unctuousness) of oil, medaha sneha (unctuosity of adipose tissue) and majja sneha (unctuosity of the marrow) gets nourished.

The medaha sneha (unctuosity of adipose tissue) nourishes snehamsha (portion of unctuosity) in the arteries and muscles that are nourished by medo dhatu (adipose tissue). Because of this the shosha (attenuation) of sira (arteries") and snayu (muscles) explained in the samprapti (pathogenesis) declines. Primarily because of Snigdha guna (unctuousness) this basti (enema) acts on the Vata which is the cardinal dosha in Pakshaghata. Apart from this it helps in the regeneration of shudha Vata (flawless Vata) in the pakwashaya (colon) which has been mentioned as the point of origin of Pakshaghata .

b. Astapana Basti (Astringent Enema) – No specific astapana basti (astringent enema) has been mentioned in Pakshaghata . A number of Vatahara basti (enemas which eliminate Vata) have been narrated in the classics. Any one of them can be administered. This basti (enema) helps in eliminating the sangakaraka padarta (choking matter) that has undergone vilayana (dissipation) through snehana krama (sequential unction) and has come to the koshta (visceral cavity) through svedana (diaphoresis). Not only that because of its Vatahara attributes (attributes of eliminating Vata), it assures prevention of repeated occlusions in the Mastishka (brain) (forestalling occlusion of the passage) and thus functions as Vata shamaka (palliative of Vata).

9. Shamana Oushadha (Palliative Medicine) –

All the aforementioned sequences mostly function in the form of shodhana (purification). Treatment will not be complete just because the dushta dosha (vitiated dosha) has been expelled. It is very important to see that this kind of dushti (vitiation) do not occur repeatedly at the point of origin (pakwashaya) and the mula adhishtana (core abode)- Mastishka (brain). Shamanoushadha (palliative medicine) accomplishes this job. For this purpose, any one or two medicines (according to requirement) listed at the terminal part of this text should be administered in proper pramana (dosage), kala (time) and with anupana (ensuing potion). This has been narrated in the relevant table. Probably most of the shamanoushadha (palliative medicines) help by eliminating the occlusive thrombus or embolism and thereby see to it that no obstruction happens in the path of Vata. This helps in adequate circulation of blood to the brain. Because of adequate blood circulation ischemia of the brain is rooted out. Mastishka (brain) is nourished, and it becomes strong. Many of the ingredients in the shamanoushadha (palliative medicine) are rakta shodhaka (purifies blood), rakta sthambaka (haemostatic) and shota hara (eliminate edema). These take care to see that no bleeding or inflammation occurs in the blood vessels of the brain. Because of this obstruction to the path of Vata do not materialize. As an example for this, Mahamanjistadi kwatha which has been listed in the table can be administered. These medicines enhance dhatvagni (medho and majja dhatvagni - metabolism of adipose and marrow tissues) and there by fortify the sira (arteries), snayu (muscles) and Mastulunga majja (marrow of the brain). To state briefly the tendency to develop vishishta vikrti (specific aberration) in one part of the Mastishka (brain) will be averted by shamanoushadha (palliative medicines). Stanika vyadhi kshmatva (localized immunity) will be enhanced. Consequently, the disposition towards khavaigunya (distortion in the passage) is forestalled.

The Samyukta karmuka prabhava (cumulative functional spell) of all the therapeutic sequences mentioned so far can be explained as follows –

Shirobasti (cephalic cumulative medicament), snehapana (oligeanous oral administration), abhyanga (unction) and other processes of abhyanga (unction) help by vilayana (dissipation) of the substances responsible for the sanga (occlusion) in the brain by undergoing sneha klinna (unctuous moisturization). The process of sveda krama (sequential diaphoresis) such as avagaha sveda (immersion diaphoresis) etc. helps in bringing the dissolved sangakaraka padarta (occlusive substance) to the koshta (visceral cavity). Virechana (laxation) and Basti (enema) help in expeditiously bringing the klinna doshas (humid doshas) moving towards the koshta (visceral cavity) into koshta (visceral cavity) and expel them. Basti functions in another way also, meaning, in the form of prakrti vighata (inherent disintegration). This has been described beforehand. When all these procedures are contemplated it appears that snehana (unction) has been given the pride of place among the shadvidhopakrama (six types of ancillary therapies).

Avastanusara Chikitsa (Stage Wise Treatment)

It is said that in Ashukari Pakshaghata (rapidly progressive Hemiplegia) associated with teevra vega (severe celerity) where signs and symptoms of vitiated Vata are inordinately present administration of Maha vata vidhwamsana rasa results in Vata shamana (alleviation of Vata) and brings about Vata samya (consonance of vata). (Ra. Ta. Sa and Si. Pra. Sam page 466).

The act of udhvahana of rakta (upward circulation of blood) enhances when Vata is aroused. There is a possibility of breach in the blood vessels because of the increased velocity in the upward flow of the blood. When the blood vessels are breached Pakshaghata can occur because of Mastishkagata rakta srava (hemorrhage in the brain). It has been said that Ekanga veer rasa is very effective in the Pakshaghata since it takes care through abating the arousal of Vata and sees to it that breaching of blood vessels do not occur by containing raktodhvahana (enhanced upward circulation of blood) (Ra. Ta. Sa and Si. Pra. Sam page 477). It has been said that Ekanga veer rasa is particularly useful in Pakshaghata seen specifically in individuals of Vata prakrti (constitution) and individuals afflicted by Upadamsha (syphilis). (Page 594).

Pakshaghata perceived in individuals of Pitta prakrti, patients of durbala hrdaya (feeble heart), medasvi (obese) and where there is accretion of Kapha and Ama (unaccomplished noxious nutrient matter) in the blood vessels Ardhanga vatari rasa is more helpful. (Ra.ta.sa.& si.pra.sam page 594)

It has been indicated to employ Tapyadi loha when the disease becomes stable after passage of initial stage of two or three days from onset of Paksaghata.

During this stage (after the first three days) Tapyadi loha is extremely effective in comparison to Ekanga veera rasa. However, it is seen to be not of much value during the jeernavasta (chronic stage).

Pancha suta rasa expeditiously ameliorates jeerna Pakshaghata (Chronic Hemiplegia).

Agnitundi vati is said to be extremely useful where there is jumjumayana (tingling), jadatha (torpidity) and gourava (heaviness), after cessation of the initial acute phase of Pakshaghata (Ra, tham.Sa. page 413).

During the jeernavasta of Pakshaghata (Chronic stage of Hemiplegia) administration of Smritisagar rasa or along with this Ekanga veer rasa for a few days' manifests extremely optimistic benefits. This drug is extremely beneficial when there is jumjumayana (tingling), jadata (torpidity), vak stabdhata (stalled speech) or vak krchrta (dysphasia). (Ra. tan.sam page 603).

Malla sindhoora is very beneficial in repeatedly occurring exacerbating Pakshaghata originating from Upadamsha (syphilis) or originating from any other cause. Ghee and honey are anupana (ensuing potions). Dose -100mg (Ra.sa.sam page 264)

Patient becomes extremely debilitated due to toxicity originating from Upadamsha (syphilis). Upadamsha surya is beneficial where Pakshaghata occurs in a patient having Aatanka (anxiety), Manasika ashanti (psychological distress), jadatva (torpidity), vichara shakti hrasa (diminution in the power of deliberation) and other symptoms. Dose: 100-150 mg with ghrta (clarified butter) (Ra.ta. sa. page 528).

During the stage of unconsciousness as well as in recent onset Pakshaghata Malla sindhoora vati can be given. Dose: 60- 100 mg twice daily with betel leaves. (ra.ta.sa.page 478)

Yogendra rasa is beneficial in the jeernavasta of Pakshaghata (Chronic Hemiplegia) due to Raktabhara vrdhi (high blood pressure), Mastishka raktavahini vidharana (breach in the blood vessels of the brain), dhamani shalyata (arterial embolism) and similar causes. This is of no use during teevravasta (acute stage). This is an excellent sowmya oushadha (placid medicine), especially in individuals with dominant Vata or dominant Pitta prakrti (constitution). This is an exceptionally divine medicine for Pakshaghata . Dose 100-150 mg (Ra.ta.sam. page 611).

Swami Krishnandaji, from his personal experience has narrated as to which medicine is more beneficial in what stage of Pakshaghata . Excluding these, it is yet to be determined by the physicians rationally employing and observing as to in which conditions which is more beneficial among the remaining medicinal formulations.

A specimen case sheet has been provided here-in-after to facilitate daily observation of the patient during the course of the treatment described so far. The data should be compiled and kept as per this.

***

MODEL CASE SHEET

Apart from compiling general data as in other case sheets, here also, the following points are to be specifically noted:

1. Desha (Geographical Region)

Desha (Geographical region)	Jangala (Arid)	Anupa (Humid)	Sadharana (ordinary)
a) Janma desha (Geographical region of birth)			
b) Vrdha desha (Geographical region of growth)			
c)Vyadhi desha (Geographical region of onset of disease)			

2. **Kala (Period)**

a) Relevant to Rtu (Season)

Varsha (Rainy)	Sharath (Autumn)	Hemantha (Late Autumn)	Shishira (Winter)	Vasanta (Spring)	Grishma (Summer)

b) Relevant to Vayaha (Age)

Balya (Childhood)	Madhyama vayasu (Middle age)	Vrdhapya (Senescent)

c) Relevant to Vyadhi (Disease)

2 months	6 months	9 months	1 Year or more

3. **Ahara and Vihara (Food and Lifestyle)**

Khara, Ruksha, Sheeta Rough Dry Cold	Ushna, Teekshna Hot Fiery	Sheeta Guru Pichila Cold Heavy Slimy

4. **Agantu (Extraneous): -** Shirobhighata (Trauma to the head), Kshata (Wounds) that are causative of excessive external bleeding, Siravyadha (Venesection)

5. **Previous Diseases That are Responsible for Mastishkagata Raktasrava (Cerebral Hemorrhage)**

Aforementioned data is essential for knowing the karana (etiology) and sadhyasadhyata (prognosis) of the disease. Relevant factors can be marked as +

6. Points Relevant to Purva Rupa (Prodromal Signs and Symptoms)

With shira shoola (headache) / without shira shoola (headache)

With chardi (vomiting)/without chardi (vomiting).

Details Relevant to Signs and Symptoms (Rupa):

I. Hasta Karma (Functions of the Hand)

a. Grhana samartya (Grasping ability): -

b. Dharana samartya (Sustaining ability): -

c. Anya vidha gati (Other types of movements)

	Anguli sandhi (Finger joints)			Manibandha sandhi (Wrist joint)			Kurpara sandhi (Elbow joint)			Kaksha (Axilla)		
Gamana karma (Movement)	Prakrta (Normal)	Madhyama (Moderate)	Avara (Inferior)	Prakrta (Normal)	Madhyama (Moderate)	Avara (Inferior)	Prakrta (Normal)	Madhyama (Moderate)	Avara (Inferior)	Prakrta (Normal)	Madhyama (Moderate)	Avara (Inferior)
a. Apakshepana (Adduction)												
b. Utkshepana (Abduction)												
c. Utkshepana (Upward lifting)												
d. Vyavartana (Rotation)												
e. Akunchana (Flexion)												
f. Prasarana (Extension)												

II. Pada karma (Functions of the Feet): -

a. Gamana Karma Samartya (Ability to Move) b. Gamana Vidhana (Gait) c. Vividha Cheshta (Varied Movements)

	Anguli (Toe)			Gulpha (Ankle)			Jaanu (Knee)			Vankshana (Pelvis)		
Gamana karma (Movement)	Prakrta (Normal)	Madhyama (Moderate)	Avara (Inferior)	Prakrta (Normal)	Madhyama (Moderate)	Avara (Inferior)	Prakrta (Normal)	Madhyama (Moderate)	Avara (Inferior)	Prakrta (Normal)	Madhyama (Moderate)	Avara (Inferior)
a. Apakshepana (Adduction)												
b. Utkshepana (Abduction)												
c. Utkshepana (Upward lifting)												
d. Vyavartana (Rotation)												
e. Akunchana (Flexion)												
f. Prasarana (Extension)												

III. Pratyavartana Kriya (Reflexes)

1. Janu pratyavartana (Knee reflex): Ksheena (weak) / Vrdha (exaggerated) /Prakrta (normal)

2. Antaradhi pratyavartana (Abdominal reflexes): Urdwa antaradhi (Upper abdominal) – Upastita (Present) / Anupastita (Absent)

Adho antaradhi (Lower abdominal)–Upastita (Present)/ Anupastita (Absent)

3. Pada pratyavartana (Foot Reflexes)

Sparsha jnana (Tactility): Upastita (Tangible) / Anupastita (Intangible)

Varna (Colour) : Prakrta (Normal) / Vikrta (Aberrant)

IV. Mamsa Peshi Stiti (Status of muscles): Krsha (Emaciated) / Katina (Hard) / Shitila (Attenuated)

V. Vak (Speech)

Stira (Stable) / Astira(Unstable)

Spashta (Distinct) / Aspashta (Indistinct)

Vyakta (Explicit) / Avyakta (Ambiguous)

VI. Twak (Skin) --

Sparsha jnana (Tactility): Upastita (Tangible)/ Anupastita (Intangible)

Varna (Colour) : Prakrta (Normal) / Vikrta (Aberrant)

Sparsha (Palpation) : Sheeta (Cold)/Ushna (Hot)/ Anushna sheeta (conventional)

Shota (Oedema): Upastita (Present)/Anupastita (Absent)

Visarpa (Erysipelas): Upastita (Present) / Anupastita (Absent)

VII. Rasa Raktavaha Srotas (Plasma and Vascular System):

Hrdroga (Cardiac ailments: Upastita (Present) / Anupastita (Absent)

Shota (Oedema): Upastita (Present) / Anupastita (Absent)

Nadi (Pulse): Yati (Rhythm), Gati (Rate): Teevra (Fast), Manda (slow), Prakrta (Normal)

Samhati (Tension), Akrti (Amplitude)–Stula (Bounding)/ Sukshma (Feeble)/Prakrta (Normal)

VIII. Annavaha srotas (Alimentary system):

Gulma (Phantom tumor): Upastita (Present)Anupastita (Absent)

Aruchi (Tastelessness): Upastita (Present) / Anupastita (Absent)

Agni (Digestive Potency): Manda (Sluggish)/ Teekshna (fiery)/ Vishama (Erratic)/ Sama (Equitable)

IX. Pureeshavaha Srotas (Excretory System):

Atisara (Diarrhoea): Upastita (Present) / Anupastita (Absent)

Malabadhata (Constipation): Upastita (Present) / Anupastita (Absent)

X. Mamsavaha Srotas (Muscular System):

Samhanana (Compactness): Uttama (superior)/ Madhyama (moderate)/ Heena (inferior)

Bhara sahatva (Weight bearing): Prakrta (Normal) / Madhyama (moderate) / Uttama (superior) / Nashta (depleted)

Samprapti Ghataka (Components of Pathogenesis) :

1. Udbhava stana (abode of origin)
2. Dosha (vitiator) – Shudha Vataja (exclusively due to Vata)/due to Vatapitta/due to Vatakapha.
3. Agni (digestive potency)
4. Ama (noxious unaccomplished nutrients)
5. Sanchara stana (domain of drift)
6. Adhishtana (abode)
7. Dushya (defiled supportive element) - Sira (artery), Snayu (muscles), Mamsa (flesh), Medas (adiposity), Majja(marrow).
8. Srotas (System /Conduits)
9. Dushti prakara (type of vitiation)
10. Vyakti stana (domain of manifestation)

Sapeksha Nidana (Differential Diagnosis)

Vyadhi vinischaya (Diagnosis): Kapha samsargaja (associated with Kapha)/ Pitta samsargaja (associated with Pitta)/ Shudha Vataja (exclusively due to Vata).

Kshayaja (due to emaciation): Bahyabhighata (External trauma) – (Doshabhighatajanya (originating from traumas due to doshas) / Abhyantara raktasravajanya (originating from internal haemorrhage).

Sadhyasadhyata (Prognosis) – Sadhya (curable)/ Krchra sadhya (difficult to cure)/ Asadhya (incurable).

Chikitsa (Treatment)

I. Nidana parivarjana (eschewal of etiology): Ruksha (rough), Khara (hard) etc. ahara vihara (food and lifestyle).

II. Samshodhana (purification):

a.Virechana (laxation) b.Basti c.Nasya

III. Samshamana

CHIKITSA PARICHARYA

THERAPEUTIC SCHEDULE

A.Virechana

1. Agnideepana (enkindle) and Sama dosha pachana (digestion of noxious unaccomplished nutrient)

Date	Vyadhi lakshana Attributes of disease Avasta lakshana Attributes of phase	Oushada medicines	Pramana Dose	Anupana Ensuing potion	Kala Time	Pathya Congenial	Parinama Result

2. Snehapana (Oleaginous oral administration): Sadyaha sneha (proximate oleaginous oral administration) / Arohana krama (Ascending sequence)

Date	Vyadhi lakshana/ Avadhi Attributes of disease/ duration	Taila/ ghrta yoga Oil/ghee formulation	Pramana Dose	Anupana Ensuing potion	Kala Time	Pathya Congenial	Parinama Result

3. Vishrama kala (Resting Period)

Date	Vyadhi avasta lakshana (Attributes of phase of illness)	Abhyangarta sneha yoga and avadhi (Oleaginous formulation for unction and duration)	Sveda prakara, dravya and avadhi (Form of diaphoresis, substance and duration)	Ahara and Anna kala (Diet and dietary timings)	Parinama (Result)

4. Virechana (Laxation)

Date	Vyadhi avasta lakshana (Attributes of phase of illness)	Abhyangarta sneha yoga and avadhi (Oleaginous formulation for unction and duration)	Virechanoushadhi (Laxative)	Pramana (Dose)	Kala (Time)	Parinama (Result)

5. Peyadi Samsarjana and Tarpana (Conciliation with thin gruel, etc and nurture)

Date	Vyadhi avasta lakshana (Attributes of Stage of illness)	Ahara vishesha (Specificity of diet)	Anna kala (Dietary timings)	Parinama (Result)

B. Basti (Enema): - Yoga (Composite)/Kala (Chronological)/ (Karma (Functional)

Date	Vyadhi avasta lakshana Attributes of phase of illness	Bastipurva abhyanga sveda and avadhi Unction preceding enema diaphoresis and duration	Basti prakara Form of Enema	Basti oushaddhi and pramana Medicament for enema and dose	Prakshepaka dravya Augmentory Substances	Kala Time	Pathya Congenial	Parinama Result

Rasa Samsarjana (Conciliation by Savoury): -

Date	Vyadhi avasta lakshana (Attributes of phase of illness)	Ahara rasa vishesha (Specificity of as dietary savoury)	Anna kala (Dietary timing)	Parinama (Result)

C. Nasya (Nasal Instillation)

Date	Vyadhi avasta lakshana (Attributes of phase of illness)	Nasya purva abhyanga and svedanarta dravya and avadhi (Unction preceding nasal instillation and substances for diaphoresis & duration)	Nasyoushadhi (Medicament for nasal instillation)	Pramana (Dose)	Kala (Time)	Pathya (Congenial)	Parinama (Result)

III. Samshamana (Palliation)

		Antaha Parimarjana (Internal Treatment)				Bahihi Parimarjana (External Treatment)					
Date	Vyadhi avasta lakshana (Attributes of phase of the illness)	Oushadhi medicament	Pramana Dose	Anupana Ensuing potion	Kala time	Abhyangarta sneha prayoga and avadhi (Oleaginous formulation for unction and duration)	Mastishkya prakara Sneha yoga avadhi (Type of therapy to brain Formulation for unction duration)	Karna puranarta snehayoga (Oleaginous formulation for instillation of ears)	Akshi tarpan-arta sneha Avadhi (Oil for nurture to the eye duration	Pathya (Congenial)	Parinama Result

1. What is the total duration of Snehapana (oleaginous oral administration)?

2. What is the total quantity of snehapana (oil administered orally)?

3. Other anushangika vichara (concomitant deliberations) on snehapana (oleaginous oral administration)

4. How many virechana (laxation) were given in total?

5. Essential points to be noted on the day virechana (laxation) was given.

6. What are the basti (enemas) given and each how many times?

7. Other noteworthy features in relation to basti (enema).

8. In Bahihi parimarjana (external treatment) what are the procedures carried out and for how many days as well as the quantity of oil used in each procedure?

The aforementioned data should be collected in order to provide a description pertaining to statistical analysis.

CHAPTER - 9

Pathya/Apathya Prakarana
Episode on Congenial/Non-congenial

Pathya (Congenial diet / activities) means taking care to see not to have any impediments in the path. Meaning taking care to see that there are no obstructions in the variety of srotas (systems) where in dhatu (supportive elements) such as rasa emanate or circulate. [Absence of impediments in the percolation through kosha bithi (cell walls), sukshma rakta vahini (capillaries of blood vessels), rakta nala (arteries), lasikavahini (lymphatic vessels etc.) of the shareera (physical body)]. Absence of impediments in these srotas (systems) ensure that the administered drug becomes easily and rapidly absorbed and its movements also becomes smooth. Pathya (congenial diet / activities) aids in the action of the drug by quick internal absorption of maximum quantity of the drug and rapid delivery to the point of khavaigunya (obstruction). Apathya (non-congenial diet /activities) causes obstruction in the srotas (systems) of dhatu (supportive elements) and not only prevents rapid absorption of the drug but also prevents adequate quantity of absorption of the drug thereby causing impairment of commensurate drug action. Therefore, it is essential to observe pathya **(congenial diet / activities)** and renounce apathya (non-congenial diet / activities). This is a common consideration in the contemplation of pathya

(congenial diet/activities) and apathya (non-congenial diet/ activities). **Employment of diet and activities that are contrary to the properties of doshas and equivalent to the properties of dhatu (supportive elements) keeping in mind samprapti ghataka (pathogenic components) comprising of doshas and dushya (defiled supportive elements) narrated for the respective illness can be termed as allegiance to pathya (congenial diet activities).**

Specific pathya/apathya **(congenial / non congenial)** have not been exclusively mentioned in the narration of Pakshaghata . However, this being a Vatavyadhi (disease of the Vata) observance of pathya **(congenial diet / activities)**, that aids in ascertaining that increased vitiation of Vata as well as vitiation of sira (arteries), snayu (muscles) and Mastulunga majja (Brain marraow) do not occur, is very much essential. Conventional pathya/apathya (congenial/non congenial) as applicable to diseases of Vata are also applicable to Pakshaghata. When and what type of pathya (congenial) is to be adhered to as well as what is apathya (non-congenial) is shown in the table. This should be followed.

Table Showing Pathya (Congenial Diet) and Apathya (Non-Congenial Diet) in Pakshaghata.

Duration	**PATHYA (Congenial Diet)**
1.During the digestive phase of Ama (Unaccomplished partially digested nutrients)	Vilepi (moderately thick rice gruel) or Odana (porridge) prepared from purana shali (old rice) – at 10 in the morning and at 8 at night accompanied with Kulatta (Horsegram) or Mudga (Greengram)

Duration	PATHYA (Congenial Diet)
	yusha (soup) prepared from tender Radish or Carrot tubers and garnished as per requirement in oil or ghee with Lashuna (Garlic), Jeera (Cumin seeds), Ela (Cardamom), Maricha (Pepper), Hingu (Asafoetida). Hot water alone should be given for drinking.
2.During the period of snehapana (Oleaginous oral administration)	Subsequent to complete digestion of the lipids consumed in the morning vilepi (moderately thick rice gruel) and yusha (soup) mentioned above may be taken garnished in the same way. Upodika (Baralla rubra), Shatapushpa (Anathemum sowa), Kakamachi (Solanum nigrum), Pudina (Mentha spicata), Methika (Mentha piperata), etc. may also be used in the yusha (soup).
3.During the vishrama kala (resting phase) after oleaginous oral administration and before shodhana (purification)	Any one of the above-mentioned foods can be taken. Dhanva mamsa rasa(soup prepared from flesh of arid animal) can be given.
4.During the period of samsarjana (conciliation) from the evening of the day of virechana (laxation).	Based upon pravara (superior) madhyama (moderate) or avara (inferior) shudhi (purification) subsequent to laxation peya (thin gruel), vilepi (moderately thick gruel), akrta

Duration	PATHYA (Congenial Diet)
	yusha (ungarnished broth) or akrta mamsa rasa (ungarnished mutton soup) can be given sequentially thrice, twice or once at the stipulated anna kala (time of consumption of food). Peya (thin gruel) and vilepi (moderately thick gruel) should be prepared from purana shali (old rice) and yusha (broth) from mudga (green gram - Phaseolus mungo).
5.Subsequent to samsarjana krama (Conciliatory sequence).	The previously narrated or the diet mentioned at item 2 should be consumed.
6.During the course of basti chikitsa (Therapeutic enema)	To be continued as mentioned above.
7. After completion of one session of Karma (functional), Kala (chronological) or Yoga (composite) basti (enema)	Rasa samsarjana krama (Sequential conciliatory procedure based on savoury) should be followed.

Important Directive: It is esential that the patient takes complete rest during the course of treatment. Anashana (fasting),Vishamashana (incompatible food), Atapa sevana (exposure to sun's heat), Vayu sevana (exposure to wind), Dhumapana (smoking), Chinta (worry), Shoka (grief), Mala mutradi vegadharana (subdue urges of defecation - urine), Diva svapna (day sleep), Ratri jagarana (staying awake at night) and Apathya ahara vihara (non- congenial food and life style) -- Patients should be informed that these are varjya (to be excluded).

Medicines That Can Be Used in Pakshaghata

Taila (Oils)

1. Anu taila (A.hri)

2. Ekadasha shatikam prasarini taila (Cha. Da)

3. Grantikadi taila (Va.Se)

4. Trtiya masha taila (Cha. Da)

5. Trshati prasarini taila (Cha.Da)

6. Dvitiya masha taila (Cha.Da)

7. Niramisha mahamasha taila (Cha.Da)

8. Bala taila (Bhai.ra)

9. Madhyama Narayana taila (Bha.pra)

9 a. Maha kukkuta mamsa taila (Bhai.ra)

10.Mahamasha taila(Cha.Da)

11.Maha Lakshminarayana taila (Yo.ra)

12.Maha Saindhavadi taila (Bha.pra)

13.Masha taila(Cha.Da)

14. Rasna Pootika taila (Yo.ra)

15.Laghu Vishagarbha taila (dvitiya) (yo.ra)

16.Vishagarbha taila (laghu)(Bhai.ra)

17. Vishatinduka taila (Ra.tha)

18.Saptaprasta brihanmasha taila(Cha.Da)

19.Sahacharadi taila (Va.Se)

Ghrita (Clarified Butter)

20.Nakuladya ghrta(Bhai.ra)

21.Brihat chagaladi ghrta (Bhai.ra)

22.Hamsadya ghrta (Bhai.ra)

Kwata (Decotions)

23. Atmaguptadi kwata (Van.se)

24.Mahamanjistadi kwata (Sha.sam)

25.Maha Rasnadi kwata (Yo.ra)

26. Masha Atmaguptadi kwata (Van.se)

27.Masha Baladi kwata (Cha.Da)

28.Ardhanga vatari rasa (Ra.ra.sa)

29.Amrita sanjeevini rasayana (Ra.yo.sa)

30.Ashtamurthy rasayana (Ra.ta)

31.Indravaruni rasa (Ra.yo.sa)

32.Ekanga veera rasa (Ra.yo.sa)

33.Kajjali (Chi.cha)

34.Kalakantaka rasa (Ra.yo.sa)

35.Pakshavata Vidwamsana rasa (Ra.Yo.Sa)

36.Pinddie rasa (Ra.tantra.sa)

37.Malla sindhura (Ra.ta.sa)

38.Yogendra rasa (Bhai.ra)

39.Rasaraja rasa (Bhai.ra)

40.Rasadi gutika (Ra.yo.sa)

41.Vata gajankusha (Bhai.ra)

42.Vata rakshasa rasa (Yo.ra)

43 Swacchanda bhairava rasa (Sha.dha)

Other Medications

44. Trayodashanga guggulu (Bha.pra)

45. Dwa trimshika guggulu (Yo.ra)

46. Visha tinduka

47. Kuchaladi yoga (Chi.cha)

48. Veera bahutee yoga. (Chi.cha)

Table Showing Taila (Oils) Used in Pakshaghata

Talia Nama Name of the Oil	Karna Purana Instillation to Ears	Nasya Instillation to Nose	Seka Fomentation	Basti Enema	Pana Oral Administration	Abhyanga Unction
Anu taila	-	+	-	-	-	+
Ekadashashatika prasarini taila	-	+	-	+	+	+
Grantikadi taila	Anirdhista (Unindicated)	=	=	=	=	=
Trtiya masha taila	-	+	+	+	-	-
Trshati prasarini taila	-	+	-	+	+	+
Dvitiya masha taila	-	-	-	+	+	+
Niramisha maha masha taila	-	-	-	+	+	+
Bala taila	+	+	+	+	-	+
Madhyama Narayana taila	-	-	-	+	+	+
Maha kukkuta mamsa taila	-	-	-	+	+	+

Talia Nama Name of the Oil	Karna Purana Instillation to Ears	Nasya Instillation to Nose	Seka Fomentation	Basti Enema	Pana Oral Administration	Abhyanga Unction
Mahamasha taila	+	+	-	+	+	+
Maha Lakshminarayana taila	+	+	+	+	+	+
Maha Saindhavadi taila	-	+	-	-	+	+
Masha taila	-	-	-	-	+	+
Rasna pootika taila	-	+	-	-	+	+
Laghu Vishagarbha taila	-	-	-	-	-	+
Vishagarbha taila	-	-	-	-	-	+
Saptaprasta brhanmasha taila	+	+	-	+	+	+
Sahacharadi taila	+	+	+	+	+	+

Taila Pramana (Quantity of Oil)

Nasya (nasal instillation) and Basti (enema) – as per classics. Karna purana (instillation of ears) – two to three drops.Abhyanga (unction) and Parishechana (sprinkle) – as required.Pana (Oral administration) with hot milk- 20-30 ml for Bhrmhana sneha (oleaginous nourishing)

Table Showing Matra (Dosage), Kala (Time) and Anupana (Ensuing Potion) of Sidha Ghrta (Formulated Ghee).

Ghrta Nama Name of the Ghee	Upayoga (Use)	Matra (Dose)	Kala (Time)	Anupana (Ensuing Potion)
1. Brihat chagaladi ghrta	Pana (oral administration)	20-30 ml	Before food twice daily	With hot water
2. Nakuladya ghrta	Pana (oral administration)	20-30 ml	Before food twice daily	With hot water
3. Hamsadya ghrta	Pana (oral administration)	20-30 ml	Before food twice daily	With hot water

Kashaya (decoction) matra, kala (dose, time) – 30-40 ml, twice daily, after food.

Rasaoushadi (mineral medicament) matra, kala (dose, time) – 125 -250 mg with honey two or three times daily after food.

S.P – The dose and time indicated above are only for guidance.

Physician can change this logically based on circumstances.

Ghataka Dravyas (Components of Formulations)

1. Akarakarabha 11 32 35
2. Arka 32
3. Arkabhakta (Suryamukhi) 11 14
4. Arkarasa 11 14
5. Agaru 1 2 8 19
6. Agnikana (Maricha) 3 15 16 24 25 31 32 34 40
7. Agnimanta (Jayantika) 9 11 14 41 43 34
8. Ajamoda 11 12 14 19
9. Ajadugdha 1 11 14
10. Ajamamsa 4
11. Arjuna 11
12. Atasi 4 11
13. Atibala 11 9
14. Ativisha 11 12 13 23 25
15. Ananta (Sariva, Yasa, Durva) 1 2 3 8 11 24
16. Apamarga (Kadabi, Kinihi) 11
17. Abbakeshara 2
18. Abhaya (Usheera) 1 2 11 14 29
19. Abhaya 11 36
20. Abhraka 31 38 39 32 42

21. Amaradaru (Devadaru, Sura) 1 2 7 8 9 10 11 14 18 19 24 25 44 9 (a)
22. Alarka (Raktarka) 14 40 47
23. Ashwata 11
24. Ashwagandha 2 5 7 8 9 10 11 14 18 21 25 27 29 39 44 9 (a)
25. Ashtavarga 20 21
26. Asana (Beejaka, Vijayasara)
27. Asavaraka (Linkopita) 2
28. Astahan (Karanja, Pootika) 11 13 24 40 49
29. Ankola 14
30. Ankoladwaya 11
31. Anghreekaraka (Angriparni, Shaliparni)
32. Antarikshajala 1 14
33. Atmagupta 4 6 9 (a) 11 13 14 18 23 24 26 27
34. Ardraka 32
35. Amaya (Kushta) 2 7 8 9 10 12 14 18 19 20 24 32 45
36. Alabu (Ikshwaku, Tumbi, Katutumbi) 11
37. Aluka 11
38. Ikshurasa 2
39. Ingudi 11
40. Indrayava 9 (a) 11 24

41. Indravaruni (Mrgadani) 8 11 24 31

42. Udumbara 11

43. Ucchata (Gunja, Jatamamsi)

44. Ela (Gopagonda) 8 9 20 21 45

45. Karkata (Madana, Karkatavisha) 2 11 41

46. Karkotaka (Bekhala) 11

47. Kakkolika (Kankola) 2

48. Kachora (Shati) 2 7 9 (a) 10 12 14 18 19 21 25 29 44

49. Katphala (Kaphala)

50. Katuka (Latakasturi, Kakkola) 2 4 14 24

51. Kartrna (Kat-trna) 2 27

52. Kadara (Shweta Khadira) 11

53. Kanaka praruha (Dhatura, Kasamarda, Kanaguggulu) 11 15 19 34 47

54. Kapiccha Beeja Kwata

55. Kapita 11 20 34 4

56. Karpura 11 21 29

57. Karamarda 11

58. Karaveera 11 15

59. Kalivrksha (Bibhitaka)

60. Kasturi 2 11

82. Kola (Badara, Chavya) 4 8 9 (a) 11 14 18 21 25 45

83. Koshamra 11

84. Kangu 11

85. Kantakari 4 9 9 (a) 24 25

86. Kanta (Kanti, Priyangu) 4 9 (a) 11 12 21

87. Kantaloha 30 31 38 42 43

88. Kunju (Kunduru, Shallaki) 2 11

89. Kharjura 11 29

90. Gaja pippali 11 44 45

91. Gadavacha 15 16

92. Gayatri (Khadira) 11 24

93. Guggulu 11 14 24 44 45

94. Guduchi 2 4 9 (a) 11 18 24 25 29 42 44

95. Gulabi (Shatadala) 11

96. Gudda 29

97. Gokanta (Gokantita, Gokshura) 4 6 7 9 10 11 19 25 29 44

98. Gopichandana 11

99. Godhuma 11

100. Gorochana 11

101. Grdramahiruha 11

102. Grshtika (Kashmarya) 11

103. Gangavati 11

104. Gandhaka 29 30 32 33 34 36 37 40 41 42 43 45

105. Gandhapatri (Patra, Ambika, Ashwanandhi)1 8

106. Gandhaprasarini 2 4 5 79 10 11

107. Grantika (Pippalimula) 2 3 5 7 9 (a) 10 14 18 45

108. Ghanasara (Putrashreni, Dantibheda) 2 11

109. Ghrta 20 22 29

110. Chaturjata 14

111. Chocha (Dalchini) 1 2 11 20

112. Chitraka 5 7 10 11 14 18 24 32 42 45

113. Choraka (Taskara) 29

114. Chandana 1 2 6 8 9 11 19 21 24 29

115. Changeri 31

116. Champeya 2 14

117. Chincha 11

118. Chagapita 34

119. Chagarasa 2 18 21

120. Chura 2

121. Jatu (Lakh)

122. Jatamamsi 2 8 9 11 14

123. Jayapala 31

124. Jala (Valaka, Hreevera) 1 21 24

125. Jalapatrika (Kamalini) 11 21

126. Jatikosha (Jatiphala) 2 12 14 39 40

127. Jatipatra 11 39

128. Jatipushpa (Malati) 21

129. Jatisasya 11

130. Jeeraka 10 12 19 21 25

131. Jeevakadi gana 2 5 6 7 8 9 (a) 10 18 21

132. Jeevanti 1 14 20 21

133. Jyotishmati 11 31

134. Janti 9 (a)

135. Tankana 30 34 41 43 47

136. Tagara 2 8 9 11 14 21

137. Tajeeraka 11

138. Tarooruha 11

139. Tavaksheera 29

140. Tamra 32 36 42

141. Taleesapatra 11 21

142. Tarkshya (Rasanjana) 2

143. Tilvaka (Lodhra) 11

144. Tila taila 1 2 3 4 5 6 7 8 9 10 11 12 13 14 15 16 17 18 19 47

145. Teekshna Loha 31 32

146. Trikatu 2 6 9 9 (a) 14 18 19 20 29 32 36 37 40 41 42 43 45

147. Trikesara 29

148. Trijataka 29

149. Triphala 2 14 20 21 24 29 32 34 45

150. Trivrit 24 44

151. Tushambu 2

152. Tuvara 44 45

153. Tuta 40

154. Tejapatra 1 8 20 45

155. Tundika 11

156. Trti (Sukshma ela) 1 2

157. Trayamana 24

158. Dadiphala 11

159. Dadhi 5 26 27

160. Dashamoola 2 5 7 8 9 (a) 10 11 14 18 20 21

161. Dadima 11 21 29

162. Daruharidra 1 2b 9 9 (a) 12 21 24 44 45

163. Draksha 11 21 29

164. Dhanvayasa 11 14 25 44 45

165. Dhananjaya 11

166. Dhatri 11 15 29 32 34 47

167. Dhanyaka 11 12 21 25 29

168. Nakulamamsa 20

169. Nakha 2 11

170. Nalika (Gandha Dravya) 2

171. Nagakeshara 1 2 11 14 32

172. Nagajihwa (Manahashila) 20 21

173. Nagabala 11

174. Nagabhasma 32

175. Nagavalli 35 36 40

176. Niyamana (Nimbi) 9 11 20 24 29

177. Nisha (Haridra) 2 9 9 (a) 11 24 29 45

178. Niva (Kadamba) 11

179. Neela kamala 1 2 12 21 29

180. Neeli 12

181. Nirgundi 11 14 32 41 43

182. Nimbuka chora 11

183. Nepathi 11

184. Padmaka 2

185. Padmakesara 1 2

207. Bahirshika (Mayurapiccha) 11

208. Bakuchi 24

209. Balayugma 29

210. Bashtika (Krishna jeeraka) 45

211. Brahmadanddi 11

212. Brahmi 11

213. Bhinddi (Manjishta) 11

214. Bidalavana 9(a) 18

215. Bilva 1 9 11

216. Beejaka (Vijayasara) 11

217. Beerbahuti 48

218. Brihati 1 9 9(a) 11 35 34

219. Bhalli 11

220. Bhanga 40

221. Bharangi 7 10 12 19 24 29

222. Bhrngaraja 11 24 34

223. Bhallataka 2 5

224. Bhupeelu 14

225. Bhutankusha Krishna nirgundi) 11

226. Bhunimba 11

227. Bhulata 22

249. Muddadaru shringa 30

250. Munitaru 11

251. Mushali (Thalamooli) 29

252. Murvamoola (Madhurasa) 11 14

253. Metika 11

254. Meshashringi 11

255. Mokha 11

256. Mouktika 38 43

257. Musta 1 2 9(a) 11 20 21 24 25 29 45

258. Manjishta 1 2 5 8 9(a) 11 14 15 18 21 24 25 41

259. Yava 4 8 14

260. Yava kshara 5 11 45

261. Yavani 9 11 40 44

262. Yashtimadhu 1 5 6 9(a) 11 12 14 18 19 20 21 29

263. Rakta agastya 11

264. Rakta kashta 11

265. Rakta jeeraka

266. Raktasara (Rakta arjuna, Rakta chandana) 112 129

267. Rajata 30 39

268. Rasa (Bola) 15

269. Rasa sindhoora 38 39

290. Vatsaka (Kutaja) 11 24

291. Varala 14

292. Varahapitta 34

293. Varishta 11

294. Varuna 14 24

295. Varusha 11

296. Vanamallika 11

297. Vasa 11 24 25 29

298. Vidhari 7 10 11

299. Vidula (Vetasa, Hijjala) 11

300. Viddanga 1 11 14 21 24 25

301. Visha (Vatsanabha)

302. Vishatindhuka 13 14 32 34 46 47

303. Visphoorjana (Kuchala) 11

304. Vridhatri 15

305. Vanga 31 32 38 39

306. Sharkara 19

307. Shakrahva (Indrayana, Indrayava) 11

308. Shanabeeja 4

309. Shatavari 1 2 7 8 9(a) 10 11 14 20 2124 25 29 44

310. Shatahva 2 4 6 7 8 9(a) 10 13 18 25 44

311. Shalyaka (Madhanaphala) 11

312. Shallaki 2 11

313. Shakotaka 2 3 24

314. Shakoruha 11

315. Shyamalata 21

316. Shalaparni 1 9 11

317. Shalmali 11 29

318. Shigru 11 14 32

319. Shilarasa 2 29

320. Shireesha 2 11

321. Shrivasa (Shreeveshtaka, Sarala) 2

322. Shukta (Kanjika) 2 5 12 15 16

323. Shudha malla 35

324. Shookashimbhi 12 27

325. Shunti 3 4 5 9(a) 11 12 23 24 25 32 34 35 44 45

326. Shringavera 5

327. Shringati 11

328. Shweta agasthya 11

329. Shweta jeeraka 7 21 27 45

330. Shaileya 2 8 9

331. Shyonaka (Tuntuka) 4 9 11

332. Sarjarasa 8

333. Sarjakshara 11 45

334. Sarshapa 14 47

335. Sarala 2 8

336. Sahachara 14 19 25

337. Sahadevi 11

338. Snigdhadaru 11

339. Sukurandda 11

340. Sugandha 11 14

341. Susurabhi (Tulasi) 11 42

342. Surabhi (Gandhasura) 1 11

343. Suvarnamukhi 11

344. Sushira 11

345. Snuhi 11

346. Soorana 11

347. Saindhava lavana 2 3 5 6 7 8 9 9(a) 10 11 12 13 15 16 18 19 22 23 26 27 45

348. Somala 30 35 37

349. Souvarcha lavana 5 9 9 (a) 18 19 45

350. Souveeram 35

351. Swarna beeja 16

352. Swarnapatra 30

353. Swarna bhasma 38 39

354. Swarnamakshika 41 43

355. Strama vrksha (Vikamkata) 11

356. Sambalu (Kanthi) 2 21

357. Hapusha 44 45

358. Haratala 30 33 40 41 43 45

359. Hareetaki 25 35 41 43

360. Hingu 7 10 14 26 27

361. Himsra (Ahimsra) 11 14

362. Hridhatri (Himavali) 11 14

363. Hemadugdha (Swarnaksheeri) 11

364. Heru (Maha Shatavari) 11

365. Hamsamamsa 22

366. Ksheera 2 5 6 7 8 9 9(a) 10 11 18 19 20 21 22

367. Ksheerakakoli 21 39

368. Putrajeevaka 11

369. Bimbeephala 11

Among the forty-nine formulations depicted above Tila taila, Saindava lavana have been used in twenty medicinal formulations. Devadaru, Aswagandha, Eranda, Kushta, Trikatu, Parada, Bala, Manjista, Rasna, Shatavari, Shunti, Ksheera-These have been used in fifteen medicinal formulations. Mareecha, Atmagupta, Kachora, Kola, Guduchi, Gokanta, Gandhaka, Pippalimoola, Chitraka, Chandana, Jeerakadi gana, Triphala, Dashamoola, Daruharidra, Punarnava, Pippali, Masha, Musta, Yeshtimadhu, Vacha, Shatapushpa – these have been used in ten medicinal formulations.

UPASAMHARA
EPILOGUE

The description pertaining to nidana (diagnosis) and chikitsa (treatment) of Pakshaghata, which can be ascribed as a dominant disease among Vatavyadhi , has so far been narrated in the right context and sequential order. When this subject is viewed 'in toto', it appears that there is sufficient scope for research apropos specific bahya nidana (external etiology) of Pakshaghata, svarupa (innate features) of majja dushti (vitiation of marrow) in samprapti (pathogenesis), potentiality of Agni karma (branding) in the treatment etc. It is also appreciable that there is scope to bring into current use Pindi rasa, Indravaruni rasa, Kalakantaka rasa, Pakshavata vidwamsa rasa, Hamsadhya ghrta, etc. which have been described in many texts, though not in prevalence and explore whether they are even more beneficial. Our attention is drawn towards abhyanga (unction) with Vishatinduka taila and Anu taila as an experimental measure.

BIBLIOGRAPHY

A. **SAMHITA GRANTA**
COMPENDIUM

1. *Charaka samhita*
2. *Sushruta samhita*
3. *Kashyapa samhita*
4. *Harita samhita*
5. *Bhela samhita*
6. *Ashtanga hridaya*
7. *Ashtanga sangraha*
8. *Sharangadhara samhita*

B. **TEEKA**

COMMENTARIES

9. *Ayurveda deepika authored by Cakrapani*
10. *Nibandha sangraha authored by Dalhana*
11. *Nyaya chandrika authored by Gayadasa*
12. *Sarvanga sundara authored by Arunadatta*
13. *Ayurveda rasayana authored by Hemadri*
14. *Commentary on Madhava nidana authored by Vijaya rakshita*

15. *Vidyotini hindi commentary authored by Sudharshana shastri*

16. *Sarvamangala commentary on Kautilya Artashastra*

C. **RASASHASTRA GRANTA BOOKS ON ALCHEMY**

17. *Rasayogasagara*

18. *Rasendrasara sangraha*

19. *Rasatarangini*

20. *Rasendra chintamani*

21. *Rasaratnakara*

22. *Rasaratna samucchaya*

D. **SANGRAHA GRANTA COMPILATIONS**

23. *Madhava nidana*

24. *Vanga sena*

25. *Basava rajeeyam*

26. *Yoga ratnakar*

27. *Bhava prakasha*

28. *Baishajya ratnavali*

E. **CHIKITSA GRANTA**

THERAPEUTIC BOOKS

29. *Chakradutta*

30. *Kalyanakaraka*

31. *Chikitsa chandrodaya*

32. *Vyadhi vijnana authored by Ashananda Pancharatna*

F. **BOOKS RELEVANT TO PATHOGENESIS**

33. *Samprapti lakshanayoho sambandha*

G. **BOOKS RELEVANT TO RACHANA AND KRIYA BOOKS RELEVANT TO ANATOMY AND PHYSIOLOGY**

34. *Ayurvediya kriya shareera*
35. *Marma vijnana*
36. *Parishadyam shabdarta shareeram*

H. **KOSHA GRANTA**
DICTIONARIES

37. *Shabdha kalpa dhruma*
38. *Shabdha stoma maha nidhi*
39. *Amarakosha*
40. *Vaidyaka shabda sindhu*
41. *Encyclopedia Britannica*
42. *Stedman's Medical Dictionary*

I. **ITIHASA GRANTA**
HISTORICAL BOOKS

43. *Vedo mei ayurveda*
44. *Ayurveda ka brihat itihasa*
45. *Ayurveda ka vaijnanika itihasa*

J. **ANYA GRANTA**
OTHER BOOKS

46. *Kautilya Artashastra*

K . **MODERN MEDICAL BOOKS**

47. *Textbook of Medicine by Harrisons*

48. *System of Medicine by Savil*

49. *Clinical Diagnosis by Golvala*

50. *Clinical Methods by Hutchinsons*

51. *Clinical Examination in Neurology, 5th edition.*

ABOUT THE AUTHOR

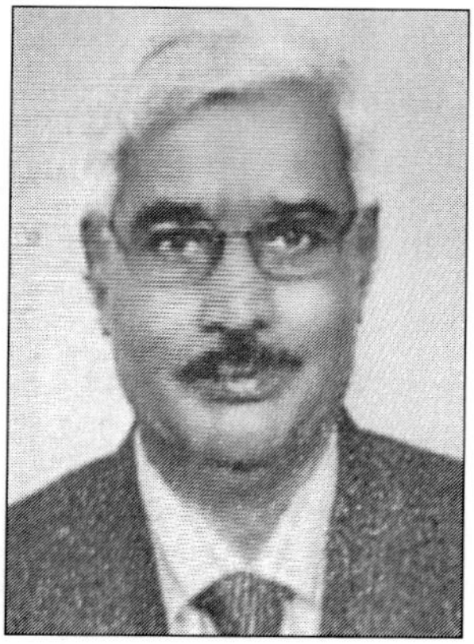

Dr. B.G.Gopinath was born in the year 1941 at the village of Barige, Soraba Taluk of Shimoga district Karnataka, to Vaidya Sri. Ganesha S Patela and Smt. Nagavenamma. His early education was at Keladi and Sagara.

He studied Ayurveda at Udupi and Postgraduate studies at Gujarat Ayurveda University, Jamnagar.

He started his carreer as Lecturer at Udupi Ayurveda College. Subsequently he joined the Government Ayurveda Medical College , Mysuru. He worked as Assisstant Professor, Professor and Head of the Department of Kayachikitsa at Mysuru and Bengaluru.

He also worked as Principal, Alva's Ayurveda Medical College Mudbidri, Karnataka; Ayurveda Medical College, Mangaluru and Mata Amrutanandamayi Ayurveda College, Kollam. He also functioned as Dean Sri Sri Ayurveda Medical College Bengaluru.

He has guided more than 35 postgraduate theses and was an examiner to all the universities in Karnataka both for undergraduate and postgraduate degree courses as well as Osmania, Kerala and NTR universities.

He was a member of the Central Council of Indian Medicine, New Delhi, Board of Studies - Bengaluru, Mysuru,

Karnataka, Mangaluru, Kuvempu and Gulbarga Universities as well as member of Board of Examiners - Bengaluru, Mysuru, Gulbarga and Kuvempu Universities.

He worked as Chairman, Ayush Health Advisory Committee, Chairman, Fourth World Ayurveda Congress and Chairman World Ayurveda Foundation Managing Committee.

He was Chairman, Board of Studies and Board of Examiners (PG) Bengaluru and Mysuru Universities.

He has presented a number of scientific papers at seminars throughout India.

He has authored a number of books including 'Clinical Methods in Ayurveda', participating in Teachers textbook writers workshop conducted by the Kerala government, Foundational Ideas of Ayurveda - in three parts,published by Council for History of Philosophy, Science and Culture , New Delhi. Philosophic Foundation of Ayurveda, Ayurveda Myths and Facts, etc.

He visited Thames Valley University London,UK as expert member of inspection committee to start an Ayurveda college at London UK.